Cambridge Studies in Oral and Literate Culture 6

THE HOLY GREYHOUND

Cambridge Studies in Oral and Literate Culture

Edited by Peter Burke and Ruth Finnegan

This series is designed to address the question of the significance of literacy in human societies: it will assess its importance for political, economic, social and cultural development, and examine how what we take to be the common functions of writing are carried out in oral cultures.

The series will be interdisciplinary, but with particular emphasis on social anthropology and social history, and will encourage cross-fertilisation between these disciplines; it will also be of interest to readers in allied fields, such as sociology, folklore and literature. Although it will include some monographs, the focus of the series will be on theoretical and comparative aspects rather than detailed description, and the books will be presented in a form accessible to non-specialist readers interested in the general subject of literacy and orality.

Books in the series
1 Nigel Philipps: *'Sijobang': Sung Narrative Poetry of West Sumatra*
2 R. W. Scribner: *For the Sake of Simple Folk: Popular Propaganda for the German Reformation*
3 Harvey J. Graff: *Literacy and Social Development in the West: A Reader*
4 Donald J. Cosentino: *Defiant Maids and Stubborn Farmers: Tradition and Invention in Mende Story Performance*
5 François Furet and Jacques Ozouf: *Reading and Writing: Literacy in France from Calvin to Jules Ferry*

This book is published as part of the joint publishing agreement established in 1977 between the Fondation de la Maison des Sciences de l'Homme and the Press Syndicate of the University of Cambridge. Titles published under this arrangement may appear in any European language, or, in the case of volumes of collected essays, in several languages.

New books will appear either as individual titles or in one of the series which the Maison des Sciences de l'Homme and the Cambridge University Press have jointly agreed to publish. All books published jointly by the Maison des Sciences de l'Homme and the Cambridge University Press will be distributed by the Press throughout the world.

Cet ouvrage est publié dans le cadre de l'accord de co-édition passé en 1977 entre la Fondation de la Maison des Sciences de l'Homme et le Press Syndicate of the University of Cambridge. Toutes les langues européennes sont admises pour les titres couverts par cet accord, et les ouvrages collectifs peuvent paraître en plusieurs langues.

Les ouvrages paraissent soit isolément, soit dans l'une des séries que la Maison des Sciences de l'Homme et Cambridge University Press ont convenu de publier ensemble. La distribution dans le monde entier des titres ainsi publiés conjointement par les deux établissements est assurée par Cambridge University Press.

THE HOLY GREYHOUND

Guinefort, healer of children since the thirteenth century

JEAN-CLAUDE SCHMITT

translated by
MARTIN THOM

CAMBRIDGE UNIVERSITY PRESS

Cambridge
London   New York   New Rochelle   Melbourne   Sydney

and

EDITIONS DE LA MAISON DES SCIENCES
DE L'HOMME

Paris

CAMBRIDGE UNIVERSITY PRESS
Cambridge, New York, Melbourne, Madrid, Cape Town, Singapore, São Paulo, Delhi

Cambridge University Press
The Edinburgh Building, Cambridge CB2 8RU, UK

With Editions de la Maison des Sciences de l'Homme
54 Boulevard Raspail, 75270 Paris Cedex 06, France

Published in the United States of America by Cambridge University Press, New York

www.cambridge.org
Information on this title: www.cambridge.org/9780521108805

Originally published in French as *Le saint lévrier: Guinefort,
guérisseur d'enfants depuis le XIIIᵉ siécle* by Flammarion, Paris, 1979,
and © Flammarion 1979

First published in English by the Maison des Sciences de l'Homme
and the Cambridge University Press 1983 as *The Holy Greyhound:
Guinefort, healer of children since the thirteenth century*.
English translation © Maison des Sciences de l'Homme and
Cambridge University Press 1983

This digitally printed version 2009

A catalogue record for this publication is available from the British Library

Library of Congress Catalogue Card Number: 81-14629

ISBN 978-0-521-24434-3 hardback
ISBN 978-0-521-10880-5 paperback

For Pauline

Ah! l'heureux temps que celui de ces fables,
Des bons démons, des esprits familiers,
Des farfadets aux mortels secourables!
On écoutait tous ces faits admirables,
Dans son manoir, près d'un large foyer:
Le père et l'oncle, et la mère, et la fille,
Et les voisins, et toute la famille,
Ouvraient l'oreille à Monsieur l'aumônier,
Qui leur faisait des contes de sorcier.
On a banni les démons et les fées;
Sous la raison, les grâces étouffés
Livrent nos coeurs à l'insipidité.
Le raisonner tristement s'accrédite:
On court, hélas! aprè la vérité:
Ah! croyez-moi, l'erreur a son mérite!

Voltaire (quoted by F. M. Luzel, in *Légendes chrétiennes de basse Bretagne*, Paris, 1881)

CONTENTS

TABLES, ILLUSTRATIONS, MAPS AND SURVEYS

Maps and surveys

ACKNOWLEDGEMENTS

This research has benefited greatly from the knowledge and generous suggestions of a large number of people. I have been greatly helped by the erudition of M. P. Cattin, Directeur des Services d'Archives for Ain, by M. J. Y. Ribault, Directeur des Services d'Archives for Cher, and by Abbé P. Armand of the Diocesan Library at Bellay. Mme Martinet, librarian of Laon, M. P. Gaché of Châteaurenard and Mme Scart of Crépy-en-Valois kindly answered questions on particular points.

I have also had very helpful discussions with numerous colleagues, often within research seminars where I was allowed to present this work. I should like, therefore, to take this opportunity of thanking Franco Alessio, Jean Batany, Michelle Bastard, Carla Casagrande, Yves Castan, Natalie Davis, Georges Duby, Daniel Fabre, Claude Gaignebet, Bronislaw Geremek, Alain Guerreau, Philippe Jontard, Lester K. Little, Ann Lombard-Jourdan, Marc Soriano, Pierre Toubert and Richard Trexler, and Miss Silvana Vecchio. I am also particularly grateful to M. J. M. Pesez and his medieval archaeology team, Françoise Piponnier and J.-M. Poisson in particular, for their continuing collaboration.

Jacques Le Goff knows better than anyone how much my research in general, and this book in particular, owes to him.

In the field I received information of great importance for my oral investigations from M. Lagrange, Mayor of Châtillon-sur-Chalaronne, M. Dagallier, Mayor of Romans, and M. Durand, Mayor of Sandrans, as well as from Mme Chevallon, Mme Goiffon, Mme Pioud, Mme Rognard, and Mme de Varax, and from M. Vacheresse and M. Vieux, of Châtillon-sur-Chalaronne.

Dr Victor Edouard of Châtillon-sur-Chalaronne, himself a historian of Saint Guinefort, unfortunately died in August 1977, before the completion of this book, which owes a great deal to him and the publication of which he awaited with interest.

Finally I must acknowledge my debt to the Centre de Recherches Historiques at the Ecole des Hautes Etudes en Sciences Sociales for material support for this research, and to the Graphics Workshop in the same institution, where several of the maps and plates for this book were made.

INTRODUCTION

The medieval church extended Christianity's influence in society considerably, at the same time strengthening what clerics of the time defined as one of its basic features, the central importance to it of the Book. This characteristic explains the rise of a learned culture which derived most of its methods of reading, interpreting and diffusing the teachings of the Bible from the classical heritage, and which led to the development of a literate, Latinate, clerical culture that helped to build the power of the church but also tended to isolate the clergy from the main body of society.

The mass of Christians did not in fact enjoy such direct access to the Scriptures or to any sort of writing. Secular culture, the culture of those whom the clergy deemed 'illiterate', i.e., those who did not know Latin (and this was often the case even at the highest levels of society),[1] was predominantly an oral, vernacular culture.

The opposition of these two cultures would seem to me to have been one of the most important features of feudal society. Their relationship was a complex one, shifting between mutual incomprehension and overt hostility, but without there ever being a complete cessation of the exchanges that such conflicts sometimes fostered. We are now beginning to acquire a better understanding of the alteration of this relationship over time, and of the reasons for it. The part played by groups seeking ideological and social advancement, for example – the petty aristocracy of knights on the secular side, the new 'intellectuals' in the church – clearly allowed quite unprecedented cultural exchanges to occur in the twelfth century, even if they were often jeopardised in subsequent years.[2]

A vast amount of historical work, however, still needs to be done. Historians are far from having identified all the elements that distinguished lay and clerical culture. For each contained an infinite variety of cultural attitudes which need to be considered in relation to the whole range of social conditions. Most important of all, we need to understand what was at stake in this opposition between cultures, to know what part it played in the functioning of feudal society, and what transformations it underwent throughout its long existence.

This book is an attempt to offer tentative answers to some of these questions. It begins with a detailed examination of a thirteenth-century document, around which I have built the book. Let me therefore introduce the document itself.

1

In 1261, a Dominican friar, Stephen of Bourbon, died at the Dominican convent at Lyons. He had spent the last years of his life in the community writing a treatise, in Latin, on the Seven Gifts of the Holy Spirit. He died without having completed his work, which has come down to us in an anonymous thirteenth-century manuscript, as well as in several later ones. For a long time the treatise remained unknown to scholars, only winning any real recognition in the hundred years since 1877, when the historian A. Lecoy de la Marche published a number of extracts from it and convincingly attributed it to Stephen of Bourbon.

The treatise is a theological commentary on the Gifts of the Holy Spirit, consisting largely of a collection of *exempla*, anecdotes, claimed to be authentic, and which were used by preachers in their sermons as edifying matter for the faithful, intended to lead them down the path of salvation. The use of *exempla* in preaching developed considerably in the course of the thirteenth and fourteenth centuries. From the first half of the thirteenth century they were assembled in collections, so as to facilitate the preacher's task. Stephen of Bourbon's work is thought to be one of the earliest collections of *exempla*.

Some of Stephen of Bourbon's *exempla* are derived from books like the Bible, or from ecclesiastical authors *(Lives of the Fathers*, Gregory the Great, etc.). Others were composed on the basis of narratives collected by Stephen of Bourbon from reliable witnesses, who gave him accounts of what they had heard or seen with their own eyes. Sometimes the oral testimony duplicates a written tradition, in which case the double transmission is taken to be an even stronger guarantee of authenticity. Thirdly, Stephen of Bourbon often composed an *exemplum* from his own experience, and it is an *exemplum* of this sort that is presented here; in it he recounts what he saw and heard in the Dombes, about forty kilometres north of Lyons.[3]

DE ADORATIONE GUINEFORTIS CANIS

Sexto dicendum est de supersticionibus contumeliosis, quarum quedam sunt contumeliose Deo, quedam proximo. Deo contumeliose sunt supersticiones que divinos honores demonibus attribuunt, vel alicui alteri creature, ut facit idolatria, et ut faciunt misere mulieres sortilege que salutem petunt adorando sambucas vel offerendo eis, contemnendo ecclesias vel sanctorum reliquias, portando ibi pueros suos vel ad formicarios vel ad res alias, ad sanitatem consequendam. [Title in the margin.]Sic faciebant nuper in diocesi Lugdunensi, ubi, cum ego predicarem contra sortilegia et confessiones audirem, multe mulieres confitebantur portasse se pueros suos apud sanctum Guinefortem. Et cum crederem esse sanctum aliquem, inquisivi, et audivi ad ultimum quod esset canis quidam leporarius, occisus per hunc modum. In diocesi Lugdunensi, prope villam monialium que dicitur Noville, in terra domini de Vilario, fuit quoddam castrum cujus dominus puerum parvulum habebat de uxore sua. Cum autem exivissent dominus et domina a domo et nutrix similiter, dimisso puero solo in cunabulis, serpens maximus intravit domum, tendens ad cunabula pueri; quod videns leporarius, qui ibi remanserat, eum velociter insequens et persequens sub cunabulo, evertit cunabula, morsibus serpentem invadens, defendentem se et canem similiter mordentem; quem ad ultimum canis occidit et a cunabulis pueri longe projecit, relinquens cunabula dicta cruentata, et terram et os suum et caput, serpentis sanguine, stans prope cunabula, male a serpente tractatus. Cum autem intrasset nutrix et hec videret, puerum credens occisum et devoratum a cane, clamavit cum maximo ejulatu; quod audiens, mater pueri similiter accurrit, idem vidit et credidit, et clamavit similiter. Similiter et miles, adveniens ibi, idem credidit, et, extrahens spatam, canem occidit. Tunc, accedentes ad puerum, invenerunt eum illesum, suaviter dormientem; inquirentes, inveniunt serpentem canis morsibus laceratum et occisum. Veritatem autem facti agnoscentes, et dolentes de hoc quod sic injuste canem occiderant sibi tam utilem, projecerunt eum in puteum qui erat ante portam castri, et acervum maximum lapidum super eum projecerunt, et arbores juxta plantaverunt in memoriam facti. Castro autem divina voluntate destructo, et terra in desertum redacta est, ab habitatore relicta. Homines autem rusticani, audientes nobile factum canis, et quomodo innocenter mortuus est pro eo de quo debuit reportare bonum, locum visitaverunt, et canem tanquam martyrem honoraverunt et pro suis infirmitatibus et necessitatibus rogaverunt, seducti a diabolo et ludificati ibi pluries, ut per hoc homines in errorem adduceret. Maxime autem mulieres que pueros habebant infirmos et morbidos ad locum eos deportabant, et in quodam castro, per leucam ab eo loco propinquo, vetulam accipiebant, que ritum agendi et demonibus offerendi et invocandi eos doceret eas, et ad locum duceret. Ad quem cum venirent, sal et quedam alia offerebant, et panniculos pueri per dumos circumstantes pendebant, et acum in lignis, que super locum creverant, figebant, et puerum nudum per foramen quod erat inter duos truncos [MS: truccos] duorum lignorum [introducebant], matre existente ex una parte et puerum tenente et proiciente novies vetule que erat ex alia parte, cum invocatione demonum adjurantes faunos, qui erant in silva Rimite, ut [MS: ubi] puerum, quem eorum dicebant, acciperent morbidum et languidum, et suum, quem secum detulerant, reportarent eis pinguem et grossum, vivum et sanum. Et, hoc facto, accipiebant matricide puerum, et ad pedem arboris super stramina cunabuli nudum puerum ponebant, et duas candelas ad mensuram pollicis in utroque capite, ab igne quem ibi detulerant, succendebant et in trunco superposito infigebant, tamdiu inde recedentes quod essent consumpte et quod nec vagientem puerum possent audire nec videre; et sic candele candentes plurimos pueros concremabant et occidebant, sicut ibidem de aliquibus reperimus. Quedam etiam retulit mihi quod, dum faunos invocasset et recederet, vidit lupum de silva exeuntem et ad puerum euntem, ad quem, nisi affectu materno miserata prevenisset, lupus vel diabolus in forma ejus eum, ut dicebat, vorasset. Si autem, redeuntes ad puerum, eum invenissent viventem, deportabant ad fluvium cujusdam aque rapide propinque, dicte Chalarone, in quo puerum novies immergebant, qui valde dura viscera habebat si evadebat nec tunc vel cito post moreretur. Ad locum autem accessimus, et populum terre convocavimus, et contra dictum predicavimus. Canem mortuum fecimus exhumari et lucum succidi, et cum eo ossa dicti canis pariter concremari, et edictum poni a dominis terre de spoliacione et redempcione eorum qui ad dictum locum pro tali causa de cetero convenirent.

Translation

On the worship of the dog Guinefort

Sixthly, I should speak of offensive superstitions, some of which are offensive to God, others to our fellow men. Offensive to God are those which honour demons or other creatures as if they were divine: it is what idolatry does, and it is what the wretched women who cast lots do, who seek salvation by worshipping elder trees or making offerings to them; scorning churches and holy relics, they take their children to these elder trees, or to anthills, or to other things in order that a cure may be effected.

This recently happened in the diocese of Lyons where, when I preached against the reading of oracles, and was hearing confession, numerous women confessed that they had taken their children to Saint Guinefort. As I thought that this was some holy person, I continued with my enquiry and finally learned that this was actually a greyhound, which had been killed in the following manner.

In the diocese of Lyons, near the enclosed nuns' village called Neuville, on the estate of the Lord of Villars, was a castle, the lord of which and his wife had a baby boy. One day, when the lord and lady had gone out of the house, and the nurse had done likewise, leaving the baby alone in the cradle, a huge serpent entered the house and approached the baby's cradle. Seeing this, the greyhound, which had remained behind, chased the serpent and, attacking it beneath the cradle, upset the cradle and bit the serpent all over, which defended itself, biting the dog equally severely. Finally, the dog killed it and threw it well away from the cradle. The cradle, the floor, the dog's mouth and head were all drenched in the serpent's blood. Although badly hurt by the serpent, the dog remained on guard beside the cradle. When the nurse came back and saw all this she thought that the dog had devoured the child, and let out a scream of misery. Hearing it the child's mother also ran up, looked, thought the same thing and screamed too. Likewise the knight, when he arrived, thought the same thing and drew his sword and killed the dog. Then, when they went closer to the baby they found it safe and sound, sleeping peacefully. Casting around for some explanation, they discovered the serpent, torn to pieces by the dog's bites, and now dead. Realising then the true facts of the matter, and deeply regretting having unjustly killed so useful a dog they threw it into a well in front of the manor door, threw a great pile of stones on top of it, and planted trees beside it, in memory of the event. Now, by divine will, the manor was destroyed and the estate, reduced to a desert,* was abandoned by its inhabitants. But the peasants, hearing of the dog's conduct and of how it had been killed, although innocent, and for a deed for which it might have expected praise, visited the place, honoured the dog as a martyr, prayed to it when they were sick or in need of something, and many there fell victim to the enticements and illusions of the devil, who in this way used to lead men into error. Above all, though, it was women with sick or weak children who took them to this place. They would go and seek out an old woman in a fortified town a league distant, and she taught them the rituals they should enact in order to make offerings to demons, and in order to invoke them, and she led them to the place. When they arrived, they would make offerings of salt and other things; they would hang their babies' swaddling-clothes on the bushes roundabout; they would drive nails into the trees which had grown in this place; they would pass the naked babies between the trunks of two trees – the mother, on one side, held the baby and threw it nine times to the old woman,

---

*The *O.E.D.* gives 'an uninhabited and uncultivated tract of country; a wilderness: a. now conceived as a desolate, barren region, waterless and treeless, and with but scanty growth of herbage. . . b. formerly more widely applied to any wild, uninhabited region, including forest-land.' It is in the latter sense that the word is employed here. *Tr.*

who was on the other side. Invoking the demons, they called upon the fauns in the forest of Rimite to take the sick, feeble child which, they said, was theirs, and to return their child that the fauns had taken away, fat and well, safe and sound.

Having done this, the infanticidal mothers took their children and laid them naked at the foot of the tree on straw from the cradle; then, using the light they had brought with them, they lit two candles, each an inch long, one on each side of the child's head and fixed them in the trunk above it. Then they withdrew until the candles had burnt out, so as not to see the child or hear him crying. Several people have told us that while the candles were burning like this they burnt and killed several babies. One woman also told me that she had just invoked the fauns and was withdrawing from the scene when she saw a wolf come out of the forest towards the baby. If maternal love had not made her feel pity and go back for him, the wolf, or as she put it, the devil in the shape of a wolf, would have devoured the baby.

When a mother returned to her child and found it still alive, she carried it out into the fast-flowing waters of a nearby river, called the Chalaronne [a tributary of the Saône], and plunged it in nine times; if it came through without dying on the spot, or shortly afterwards, it had a very strong constitution.

We went to this place, we called together all the people on the estate, and we preached against everything that had been said. We had the dead dog disinterred, and the sacred wood cut down and burnt, along with the remains of the dog. And I had an edict passed by the lords of the estate, warning that anyone going thenceforth to that place for any such reason would be liable to have his possessions seized and then sold.

Although this document has been available to scholars for a hundred years it has never previously been fully studied. Graus, the great historian of early medieval hagiography, mentions it in a footnote, but his book, outstanding though it is, is grounded in a set of concerns and a methodology which prevents him from making fuller use of it. Most of the references to this document are by folklorists; some, notably Baring-Gould in England and Saintyves in France, are interested exclusively in the narrative of the dog's death, which they compare to similar narratives in medieval literature or in more recent popular literature, and some literary historians, Gaston Paris in particular, have shared this approach. Other folklorists have concentrated their attention upon the child-healing rite, so as to demonstrate the antiquity of ritual practices still surviving in the countryside. Finally, local historians have seen the text as a picturesque illustration of the 'primitivism' which has long been attributed to the inhabitants of the Dombes. Very few have sought to give this document the thorough investigation that it deserves.[4]

One can perhaps account for this silence, and for the inadequate treatment that this document has received in the last hundred years, in terms of a fundamentally ideological reluctance to admit that such a cult could have existed. One could also invoke the general positivism of the period, and the lack of contact between disciplines. This new attempt at an interpretation has not come about by chance, however, but is the outcome of a collective enquiry into the literature of *exempla*, the narrative genre to which this document belongs.[5] This enquiry is itself part of a broad current of research into 'popular literature', 'oral traditions', 'popular culture', 'popular religion' and so on. I do not propose, however, to survey the various and often contradictory approaches that these expressions cover,[6] nor even to situate my own work in relation to them. My approach and methodology will become clear as I proceed with the analysis of the text. Meanwhile, I shall simply set out the main questions that the text raises, and try to explain how I think one might answer them.

There is one question that is in urgent need of an answer. It concerns the relationship between the two cultures, one of which is literate, Latinate, urban, clerical, responsible for Christian orthodoxy, drawing its strength from its powers of temporal and spiritual coercion, and which produced this text, the other of which is popular (in the limited, sociological sense of the word), oral, vernacular, peasant, secular, Christian also (although in a different sense), and which, in the text, is the object of both a description and a repression. I shall follow the conventional usage, and call the former 'learned culture' and the latter 'folk culture'. (The advantage of this latter term is that it avoids the ambiguities attached to the term 'popular', although it admits those attached to the term 'folk', or to 'folklore'.) However, regardless of the customary use of the term ('folk'/'folklore'), my choice of 'folk culture' clearly situates the present work within a scientific anthropological perspective.

My second question ought properly to come first, for it is one that is invariably raised when one conducts research based upon documents from the past. If one considers the beliefs and practices described in the text, which are clearly quite startling, to be too startling to 'be true', and if one supposes that Stephen of Bourbon, for instance, misunderstood what he was told and that peasants could never, even as long ago as that, have venerated the memory of a dog and 'canonised' it,[7] one may as well abandon one's research there and then. If, on the other hand, one thinks that there may be a meaning to it all, and that the document ought to be taken seriously, then that clearly provides a tremendous opportunity for a new approach to medieval history. Unexpected forms of mass culture may then come to light, which have hitherto been obscured by traditional hagiography's mode of presentation of a church culture whose heir, after all, it is.

This is indeed what I would hope to achieve. But new concerns and new approaches require a new methodology. Traditional methods, as I have said, have been incapable of solving the problems presented by a document of this sort. Traditional medieval history is for the most part unaware of the oral tradition, literary history is too concerned with a narrative's formal and aesthetic characteristics, religious history is too inclined to view 'popular religion' as a dim, deviant and irrational reflection of the religion of the élites, while folklorists all too often lack a historical perspective.

But the encounter between history and anthropology would now seem to permit a new methodology and a new set of concerns. Both disciplines may benefit from this encounter. The ethnology of 'complex societies' and the anthropology of 'preliterate' societies offer the historian not merely information but new methods (structural analysis, in particular) and a clearer perception of the problems of structure, and of the possibilities of comparison. But historians need to assimilate these borrowings whilst retaining the familiar analytical techniques and requirements of the chronological dimension (history's defining feature, albeit one that the other humane sciences are now adopting), without which it is impossible to study social structures and their transformations.

These are the circumstances in which 'historical anthropology' or 'ethnohistory' are taking shape. This book will, I trust, assist the emergence of these new disciplines.

PART I

The inquisitor

The above text is of great interest for the understanding of thirteenth century folk culture, and if I have presented it so unceremoniously at the start of the book it is so that it might have the same impact on the reader as it did on me when I first read it. Such documents are extremely rare for this period.

It would, however, be wrong to treat it as direct evidence of folk culture. It is primarily a document from the learned culture, written in Latin by a cleric, produced in circumstances in which folklore was being brutally repressed, and it was ultimately intended to be used, in the form of an *exemplum*, as an argument against 'superstitions'.

1

STEPHEN OF BOURBON

Very little is known about Stephen of Bourbon, author of the treatise from which the *exemplum* is taken, beyond the few pieces of information to be gathered from the work itself and the details given us by Bernard Gui, the Dominican inquisitor, at the beginning of the fourteenth century.[1] He was born at Belleville-sur-Saône in about 1180 (his name merely indicating geographical origin rather than membership of the family that has since become famous). He began his studies at the cathedral school of Saint Vincent at Mâcon, where he was a *puer*, a scholar. At the beginning of the thirteenth century, in around 1217, when he was about twenty-five years old, he was a student (*juvenis, studiens, scholaris*) in the Parisian schools from which the University of Paris was created in 1231.

He joined the Dominicans some time after their arrival in Paris in 1217, and the foundation of the House of Jacobins the following year, entering the order by 1223 at the latest, and completing his theological training there. Yet the only convent to which he would seem to have been attached is the one in Lyons, founded in 1218. He was there in 1223, having returned to the region where he was born, and he died there in 1262. But he did not properly retire from the world until the end of his life, when he wrote his book.

In the interim he travelled widely in what is now the Rhône–Alps region, going as far afield as Burgundy, Champagne, the Jura, the Alps, the region of Valence, the Auvergne, Forez, and even to Roussillon. In the course of these journeys, Stephen of Bourbon collected various eyewitness accounts and had encounters himself which provided him with material for many of his *exempla*.

When Stephen of Bourbon recounts one of these personal experiences he very often indicates that it happened to him in his capacity as a preacher: 'Cum ego predicarem . . .', 'When I was preaching . . .'. It is immediately clear that he was not a regular preacher restricted to an often narrow preaching area (*praedicatio*) or to the collection points (*termini*) of a single convent. His activities appear more like those of a preacher-general. These first appeared in 1228, and were chosen for their competence in theology (they were required to have studied for at least three years, rather than for the ordinary friars' one year) and for their skill as preachers. They were appointed by the provincial chapter, of which they then became full members.[2] Yet Stephen of Bourbon travelled and preached well beyond the boundaries of the Dominican province of France to which the House of

Lyons belonged, and he never refers to himself as *predicator generalis*. Only the status of inquisitor, granted by pontifical mandate, could justify such extensive travelling, and Stephen of Bourbon confirms this himself in the book.

The office of inquisitor must have been conferred on him in about 1235, in the diocese of Valence, where the Waldensian heresy (which had appeared half a century earlier in Lyons) was rife. He was also involved in the trial of the heretics of Mont-Aimé in Champagne, sent for torture by Robert le Bougre. He was one of the first inquisitors, appointed only three years after Pope Gregory IX had entrusted the duties of the inquisition to the Dominican order. The office involved specialised jurisdiction in heresy investigations and had at first been held by bishops. Then at the end of the twelfth century, the apostolic see resumed control of it once more and delegated its powers to the pontifical legates, who had various successes. In 1232 and 1238 the Pope conferred these powers upon the Dominicans, and then upon the Franciscans, through the person of their master-general. This was the birth of the Inquisition. The heads of the various orders in their turn delegated their powers to the masters provincial who delegated them to friar inquisitors, who, however, carried out their duties in the name of the Pope himself, or *mandato apostolico*, as Stephen of Bourbon says of his own situation.

His inquisitorial duties explain why he travelled so constantly, and they also account for his interest in rural areas and their inhabitants. At first sight it might seem paradoxical for a member of a mendicant order whose main mission was the apostolate in towns and cities, who had received his theological education as a friar in Paris and who was attached to the House of Lyons, to spend so much time in the countryside. But, in his pursuit of heretics, he was forever tramping across it. He would visit isolated manors, towns and villages, and in the course of his journeys he would learn many other things as well.

His main informants were country curés, who told him of any irregularities in their flocks, and these furnished material for his *exempla*. This was particularly the case in the Rhône–Alps region, which he knew well, for he had been born there. Compared with, say, the Midi there was very little urbanisation there, especially to the East of the Saône. It was therefore rare for the mendicant orders, who preferred towns, to establish houses there. By the mid thirteenth century there were religious houses only at Lyons (Franciscans and Dominicans), Mâcon (Franciscans and Dominicans) and Villefranche (Franciscans). To the East of the Saône the whole of what is now the *département* of Ain, which includes the Dombes, had no mendicant settlement until the Carmelites founded a house in 1343.[3] This 'mendicant desert' may perhaps have forced the friars to compensate for the somewhat sparse distribution of convents by more intensive rural preaching.

Most importantly they needed to respond in kind to the propaganda of their main adversaries in the region, the Waldensians, who went from village to village preaching their doctrine.[4] It was perhaps on one of his inquisitorial circuits of the Dombes that Stephen of Bourbon came across the strange cult of Saint Guinefort.

2

ON 'SUPERSTITION'

Stephen of Bourbon's work was to have been in seven sections, each one being named after one of the Seven Gifts of the Holy Spirit: the Gifts of Fear, Piety, Knowledge, Fortitude, Counsel, Understanding and Wisdom. But death overtook him before he had completed the section devoted to the Gift of Counsel or made a start on the last two sections.

Reflections on the Seven Gifts of the Holy Spirit derived from the teachings of Saint Augustine and were at the centre of scholastic philosophy in the thirteenth century. Two authors close to Stephen of Bourbon, both also attached to the House of Lyons, chose to write on the same topic: Humbert of Romans, who later became master-general, wrote a treatise on the Gift of Fear (*De dono timoris*) which was largely inspired by the corresponding section in Stephen of Bourbon's work, and William of Perraud wrote another *Treatise on the Seven Gifts of the Holy Spirit*.

Reflections on this subject were a special concern of Dominican theologians, the crowning achievement in this genre being the work of the most famous of all of them, Saint Thomas Aquinas (who died in 1276), who sought to define the difference between virtues, which cause Christians to act *modo humano*, through their human qualities, and Gifts, which, coming from God, are superior to virtues and which enable them to act *ultra modum humanum*, in a superhuman manner.[1]

Stephen of Bourbon did not know of the teachings of Aquinas, who was his exact contemporary. His own theological reflections are less far-reaching, but then his purpose was not the same. His perspective was a pastoral rather than a speculative one, and he was chiefly concerned to show by means of concrete *exempla* which moral rules derived from which Gift. In the fourth section, however, the Gift of Strength (from which the Guinefort text comes), there is an echo of contemporary theological speculation regarding the Gifts of the Holy Spirit, the Virtues and the Vices. In fact the author recalls that the Gift of Strength encourages us to repel the Seven Vices 'in a manly fashion'[2] and then goes on to use the Vices as headings for the seven subdivisions (*tituli*) of the fourth section: Pride (*Superbia*), Envy (*Invidia*), Anger (*Ira*), Sloth (*Acedia*), Avarice (*Avaricia*), Lust (*Luxuria*), and Gluttony (*Gula*).

Each of these *tituli* is divided into chapters (*capitulae*) which are each subdivided into seven paragraphs. This is the scholastic mania for classification taken almost to the point of caricature, and Stephen of

Bourbon is sometimes snared by his own *schemae*, and finds himself incapable of furnishing any content for his *a priori* subdivisions. Remembering the function of a work of this nature, however, such classifications would help a preacher looking for *exempla* to find his way around a very dense manuscript text, and help him remember the logical sequence of the narratives. These classification systems were principally mnemotechnic devices.

The first Vice that the Gift of Strength helps us repel is Pride. The traditional view, that Pride was 'the head and source of all the Vices', had been considerably undermined by recent social changes,[3] but Stephen of Bourbon adheres to it nonetheless.

The sixteen chapters on Pride can be divided into two distinct groups. The first eight are concerned with individual aspects of Pride: vainglory, vanity, ambition, hypocrisy etc. The eight others deal with the social implications of the Vice of Pride, which is thought to stir up insubordination to the laws of the church: the source of disobedience (*inobediencia*), rebellion (*contumacia*), irreverence and sacrilege against persons (*irreverencia et sacrilegium personale*), sacrilege against holy places (*sacrilegium locale*), violation of saints' days (*sacrorum festorum violacio*), presumption (*praesumpcio*), heresy (*haeresis*), and finally superstition (*superstitio*).

Superstitions therefore come last, after heresy but separate from it, among the manifestations of overt hostility to God, his church and religion. The Guinefort text is in this last chapter. What, then, does Stephen of Bourbon mean by 'superstition'?

Even in Roman times the word *superstitio* was used – in opposition to *religio*, which meant religious scruple – to signify a degraded and perverted form of religion.[4] The Church Fathers, Isidore of Seville in particular,[5] confirmed this unfavourable judgement by linking superstition with heresy, schism and paganism, whereas in the Middle Ages superstitions were termed 'vain, superfluous and redundant observances' (*vacua, superflua, superinstituta*).[6] Lucretius's etymology of the word, which suggests that superstitions are concerned with 'superior' things, matters 'celestial and divine', was rejected by Isidore, and by everyone thereafter, with understandable vigour ('Lucretius male dicit' . . .).

The idea that superstitions were 'observances' which had survived from another age, and for which they were a kind of evidence (*superstites*), and the gradual absorption of folk practices and pagan survivals into the church's calendar, finally enabled it to rule that any folk practices which deviated from its standards were superstitious.

In this sense, the word *superstitio* in the twelfth and thirteenth centuries designates a category in learned or university thought. It is worth noting, moreover, that the traditionally adverse comments of the clergy were offset by the somewhat ambivalent curiosity of those intellectuals who were attracted by the *mirabilia* of oral tradition – such as Geoffrey of Monmouth or Gervase of Tilbury – or by the practical efficacy of the folk culture. Thus, around 1265 or 1267, the Franciscan Roger Bacon (who was, admittedly, to abandon the university milieu) speaks with some sympathy of Peter of Maricourt, a 'master of experiments' who was anxious to know everything and 'took note even of the experiments, the *sortileges*** and the songs of old women and of all the magicians'.[7]

But most of the clergy condemned superstitions as belonging to demonic forces. The best-known authorities, such as John of Salisbury (d. 1182), in his *Polycraticus*, or William of Auvergne (1180–1249), in *De universo,*[8] enquired as to the status of superstitions. They had to be defined and classified so that they might be combated more effectively. Scholastic philosophy made some remarkable achievements in this respect, the greatest, again, being in Aquinas's *Summa*. Stephen of Bourbon, his contemporary, was too 'provincial' and too absorbed in other tasks to have benefited from the teachings of this Parisian authority, as we have seen, and never refers to him in his writings. Their approaches are often similar, but Stephen of Bourbon's stops short of the Thomist synthesis. On some points he is clearly pre-Aquinan, as for example on the subject of witchcraft, where he wholly accepts the traditional view that attributes its consequences to 'illusions of the devil', whereas from Aquinas onwards the opposite idea gains credence, namely, that it involves real women who gather at night, thus opening the way to the massive persecutions at the close of the Middle Ages.[9]

Stephen of Bourbon divides superstitions into 'divinations, incantations, sortileges, and the various tricks of demons'. All of these practices are described as 'vain worship' which, like 'vainglory', stems from *Superbia*, the vice of Pride, which is the opposite of *Humilitas*, the humility of the true Christian towards God. And, as the introduction to the *exemplum* shows, it is an attitude that leads to the contempt in which proud men hold both God and their neighbours, in imitation of the demons who were angels before pride caused their fall. The influence of Saint Augustine is quite apparent here.[10]

With superstition, then, God is the victim and the devil the beneficiary; the whole of this section is dedicated, as it were, to the devil. His power is manifested in superstition, its only purpose being to seduce (*seductio*) and to mislead (*ludificatio*). Inasmuch as it can only operate with God's permission, and is therefore checked by the exorcisms performed by

---

*The *O.E.D.* gives 'the practice of casting lots in order to decide something or forecast the future; divination based on this procedure or performed in some other way', and the word is used in this sense by Keith Thomas in *Religion and the Decline of Magic* (London, 1971). *Tr.*

bishops and by the force of the sacraments, it is a limited power, but nevertheless a real one.

The devil can assume a human form (*transmutatio, transfiguratio*) so as, for example, to appear to someone in the guise of a neighbour who would then strive to kill small children; by means of this stratagem the devil seeks to bring innocent people into disrepute, and a careful investigation is required in order to show that there has been diabolic deception and that the neighbours could not possibly have acted in such a manner.

The devil often works through the intermediary of 'soothsayers'. Stephen of Bourbon does not doubt their capabilities, so long as the devil is acting through them. For example, when one of them is using a sword (*spata*) to discover who is responsible for a theft, the devil causes the face of an innocent person to appear to him. The nocturnal invocations of a woman soothsayer (*divina*) cause the devil to rise up in the shape of a 'terrifying shadow' which starts to speak. The invocations another makes on behalf of a barren woman cause her to conceive a child whose diabolic nature is revealed at its baptism.

In order for these men and, in particular, these women (*divina, vetula, sortilega*) to achieve successful results it is necessary for the devil to act through them. In fact, as far as Stephen of Bourbon is concerned, the devil is really solely responsible. The soothsayers, left to their own devices, are nothing but laughable charlatans. He ridicules them continually – the augurs who claim to be able to read omens in the songs of birds (crows and cuckoos) only succeed in convincing the stupid; soothsayers who maintain that they know everything about some person, or that they can locate a stolen object or change water into wine, actually employ stratagems designed to mislead the credulous. It is not certain, moreover, that such opinions were the exclusive monopoly of the learned culture, for the soothsayers' regular clients were probably quite capable of distinguishing between those who had recognised powers and the general run of imposters.[11] The difference is that Bourbon argues, on the basis of a few instances of fraudulent practice, that all superstition is trickery. Whether he grants that a diabolic result has been achieved or whether an ordinary charlatan has simply taken advantage of a credulous woman, it is all trickery and is opposed to the truth, which belongs exclusively to God and to the church.

To understand Bourbon's attitude, the *exemplum* needs to be seen in the context of learned culture. The *exemplum* is an illustration of the devil's power to mislead. It was the devil who was responsible for starting the pilgrimage by 'his enticements and illusions . . . [which] led men into error'.

But the devil is not solely responsible. Although in other places Stephen of Bourbon simply denounced the devil's tricks, here he is bound to take human responsibility into account. For this is a rite in which women consciously ask the devil's help. They make offerings to him and, most crucially, they *invoke* him in rituals; it is a *vetula*, an old woman and in actual fact a witch, who teaches the mothers the formulae to use; these women then invoke the 'fauns' by passing the child between the trees. Bourbon mentions invocation a third time when the wolf, which is treated as substitute for the devil, comes out of the forest. There is more than what Aquinas would call a 'tacit pact' between the women and the devil: they do not just do things that make the intervention of the devil possible, they explicitly seek his aid, making a 'distinct pact' with him, which is a sign of the gravest of superstitions, idolatry.

Stephen of Bourbon does in fact link the practices he denounces with idolatry. Idolatry, in the Augustinian tradition, is the worst superstition, and Aquinas still regards it as the most serious. According to him it consists 'in improperly according divine honour to a creature'.[12] These are the very terms that Stephen of Bourbon employs in his introduction to the *exemplum*, and the attitude of the mothers seems to fit the definition, both when they invoke the demons – creatures of God – and when they hope for a cure from the tomb of a dog, a creature whose diabolic nature Stephen of Bourbon never doubts. There are two other *exempla* close to this one in the collection which deal with similar themes, one depicting the diabolic pack of hounds of the *mesnie Hellequin** and the other the appearance of the devil in the shape of a black dog in a village in the Forez region.[13]

Another category is mingled with idolatry here, namely, the casting of lots. It was against sortileges that Stephen of Bourbon had come to preach, and he denounces the 'wretched women who cast lots'. The word 'lot' (*sort*) means primarily a process of divination. Divination allows an action to be taken in the certain knowledge that it will turn out well. The practice can hardly be reconciled with Christian thought, since it presupposes a desire to know God's plan in advance, perhaps to modify it but certainly to deprive him of control over the future. There are some scriptural texts, however, that could be read as condoning the use of lots, and theologians were often hesitant to condemn them outright, until the growing persecution of witches finally put paid to this hesitation and caused them to condemn, under the same heading, sortilege, divination and the invocation of demons.[14] All three offences occur, in quick succession, in the final part of the curative rite described by Stephen of Bourbon.

There is, finally, one other form of superstition involved, which Aquinas called 'the superstition of the improper worship of the true God', i.e., Christian worship put to wrong use. To the inquisitor, the rite performed by the mothers appears a sacrilegious mockery of true pilgrimage, and

---

**Mesnie Hellequin* was the French and Norman term, from the twelfth century onwards, for the Wild Hunt. Hellequin was the name of the phantasmal leader of this troop of ghosts. *Tr.*

venerating a dog as 'martyr' seems an offence against the worship of the saints. This is mainly because these women 'scorn the churches and holy relics' which for Stephen of Bourbon are all that is efficacious, in favour of a kind of worship which is superstitious – which means that in his eyes it is essentially vain and useless – but he is also angry because he had originally hoped to discover a 'true' saint whose existence was hitherto unknown to him.

In actual fact, any attempt by peasants to define the criteria of sanctity (even had the saint been a man) would have appeared subversive to Stephen of Bourbon. For a century or more it had been the Pope's task, and his alone, to institute the canonisation of saints. This entailed a long and strictly controlled 'process of canonisation', during which a commission composed of three cardinals made a detailed enquiry and the responses of trustworthy witnesses were entered in writing and rigorously examined.[15] The worship of Saint Guinefort was not therefore simply an indication of the ignorance or sheer presumptuousness of the peasants, for it was also, to a Dominican, a challenge to the highest authorities of the church.

As the West became Christianised and popular forms of Christian worship developed, the third kind of superstition, that of the 'improper worship of the true God', must have assumed greater importance. Saint Augustine had been aware of this third kind, but he gave priority to combating the first kind of superstition, idolatry, i.e., the worship of idols and pagan gods which the Church Fathers and conciliar decrees treated as demons. As paganism receded, the absorption of Christian practices into folk culture drew the clergy's attention increasingly to 'the improper worship of the true God'. The *exempla* provide ample evidence for this, and of superstitions concerning the eucharistic host in particular. Aquinas accords this type of superstition the greatest importance, giving it precedence over 'idolatry', 'divination', and 'reading lots'. Idolatry still remains the most serious of these, but no longer attracts the most attention.

With relatively less attention being paid to idolatry, its place in the social order shifted. Originally it came from *paganitas*, and it is still linked to the 'peasantry'. There is a plethora of texts that describe the countryside as the repository of pagan practices. William of Auvergne speaks of the 'ancient idolatry' (*antiqua idolatria*) and the 'relics of ancient superstition' (*reliquiae superstitionis antiquae*) still rife in rural areas.[16]

Stephen of Bourbon is less explicit on this point, but his vocabulary shows the same conceptions to be at work: when he uses the words *lucus* (sacred wood) or *faunus* (faun) he is referring specifically to the religious vocabulary of ancient Rome. The word *lucus* used in the sense of 'sacred wood' is rare in the medieval vocabulary, where it is commonly used to mean 'wood', the material.[17] The word is frequently found in its religious sense, however, in classical Latin.[18] It is still used in this sense in the repeated condemnations of German pagan practices from the eighth to the eleventh century; Tacitus had previously asserted that the Germans gave the names of gods to their sacred woods (*luci ac nemora*); in his campaigns against the Saxons Charlemagne had several *luci* destroyed, the most famous of which was Irmensul; and around 1074 to 1083 Adam of Bremen asserts that the Suevians had a *lucus* in which they hung the corpses of dogs, horses and men that had been sacrificed to their gods.[19]

Stephen of Bourbon was probably not familiar with all of these examples, but it is clear that the word was closely associated, in the vocabulary of the clergy, with ancient paganism and its supposed survivals. By applying it to a cult site that he has suppressed, Stephen of Bourbon gives every indication of having regarded these superstitious practices as survivals from the idolatry of ancient times.

The allusion to fauns bears out this hypothesis. Faunus was a divinity of the whole countryside, more or less distinct from Silvanus, who was the god of the woods alone.[20] His feast was kept on 15 February, at the time of the Lupercalia, a word whose etymology is still obscure but which has some sort of connection with the wolf (*lupus*). It is interesting that the aggression of the wolf should be linked in the text with the activities of the fauns, for both creatures are diabolic and come out from the forest.

The mythographers of the late classical period tried to derive *faunus* from the root form of the verb *fari*, to speak publicly and religiously, as also from another derivative, *fatuus*, a fool. *Faunus* or *fatuus* were also given consorts, *Fauna* or *Fatua*, presented as their wives (*uxor eius*) and associated with *Fata*, goddess of fate (*fatum*), from whose name the French *fée* (fairy), first recorded in the twelfth century, is derived. This whole semantic area is an extremely rich field of investigation, for in it the truths of a 'mad' speech are mingled with the murky powers of prophecy. This combination may well recur in history in both the exaltation of 'holy madness', such as is found in the guise of 'God's fool',[21] in the East in particular, and in the mixture of attraction and fear provoked by those fairies ('good' or 'bad') which the clergy include under the heading of demonic.

The spread of Christianity demanded that any divine speech that was not that of the true God and controlled by the church be condemned, and the clergy were not slow to define as demons all those 'choruses of old people' who, according to Martianus Capella, 'inhabit the forests, lakes, springs and rivers, and go under a variety of names: *Fanes, Fauni, Fones, Satyri, Nymphae* and *Fatuae*, or again *Fanae*, but have in common the gift of prophecy'.[22]

From the late classical period onward, fauns were sometimes taken to be demons,[23] but the real turning point came when the Church Fathers included fauns in the Christian demonological system. It was in relation to fauns that Saint Augustine drew up what Jacques Le Goff has called the 'birth certificate of incubi in the Middle Ages':[24] 'the people call the spirits of the woods and the fauns incubi',[25] i.e., demons of the male sex, as opposed to 'succubi'. This Augustinian tradition spans the Middle Ages from Isidore of Seville [26] to William of Auvergne, who describes a faun as 'the son of an incubus'.[27] There is nothing anodyne about the choice of words here, for they indicate quite clearly a double response to a then quite heated debate about the nature of demons. William of Auvergne's attitude in the first half of the thirteenth century was that incubi could beget children, and therefore had a material reality and were not 'pure spirits'. On this last point he is critical, as his formula implies, of the sceptical attitude of Gervase of Tilbury in the previous century, who had been reluctant to grant fauns the body of a 'sylvan animal' like the one classically described in the *Life of Saint Anthony* as 'a dwarf-like creature with a hooked nose, horns growing from his forehead and goat's feet'.[28] Saint Jerome uses the same image in the *Life of Saint Paul,*[29] and it was commonplace up until the time of William of Auvergne.

William of Auvergne also describes the faun's behaviour, which lends credence to the etymology of its name. *Faunus* comes from *fatuus*, mad, and he gives the French equivalent *folet*, a folk term which is still used nowadays for imaginary and malicious beings. *Follets* (goblins) play tricks on men and upset animals, appear unexpectedly and vanish just as suddenly, make a rumpus in the night, lead travellers astray on the moors and then take to the rocks (the rock of Lutin, at Noirmoutier) or hide in a dolmen.[30] William of Auvergne derives the entire psychology of the faun from the word *folet*: 'He retains little of the light of natural wisdom . . . The most stupid threats, even meaningless ones, terrify him, and acting out of fear of the threats that are piled against him, he obeys the orders of men.' But his madness also sends him into fits of tremendous anger.

We can now see more clearly what Stephen of Bourbon means when he speaks of 'fauns': incubi, therefore male, born perhaps of a union between a demon and a woman, avatars of pagan divinities, temperamentally unstable, veering between docility and fear and sometimes becoming violently angry, but also ready to respond to the invocations of man. It also helps to explain how fauns, horned demons with goat's feet, could by association come to be used as attendant figures of the great goat of the sabbaths.[31]

Stephen of Bourbon's vocabulary shows quite clearly that he thought of himself as combating the survivals of paganism, and his actions, too, as he describes them, seem partly to follow ancient patterns dating from the time when paganism really was the church's main target. The same is also to some extent true of the final calling together of the 'people' to witness the destruction of the cult site. Saint Marcellus of Paris, according to his biographer Fortunatus (*c.* 600), 'called the people together' as he joined battle with the dragon which was terrorising the town.[32] The *Canon episcopi*, which was the main juridical weapon in the fight against superstition from the tenth to the thirteenth century, prescribed that priests should denounce 'pagan error' before 'all the people' assembled in the church.[33] Finally, after the revival of heresy in the West, Gerard of Cambrai in 1025 preached a 'general sermon to the people' against the heretics.[34]

But Stephen of Bourbon's 'calling the people together' ought also to be considered in another context and need not necessarily have such an archaistic significance. The same cannot be said for the destruction of the cult site, for in this respect Stephen of Bourbon acts exactly like a bishop or saint of the early Middle Ages.

Early medieval hagiography provides plentiful evidence of 'sacred trees' destroyed with savage zeal by missionary saints and holy bishops.[35] It was in this manner that Saint Amator set Germanus of Auxerre on the path to conversion and to sainthood: Germanus, who was a great hunter, used to hang the heads of the game he had killed on the branches of trees. One day the bishop took advantage of his absence to cut down 'the sacrilegious tree, stump and all, and, in order that the unbelievers might not retain any memory of it, he had it burned immediately'.[36]

Charlemagne's ravages against the Saxons were inspired by the same model: 'He destroyed their temple and their sacred wood, Irmensul, which was so renowned.' And Eigil (d.822) adds of this same expedition that 'they cut down the sacred woods and built holy basilicas'.[37]

The famous *Decretum* of Bishop Burchard of Worms at the beginning of the eleventh century, recapitulating the decision of an earlier council, drew the bishops' attention to 'trees consecrated to demons that the people worship, and which they venerate to such a degree that they do not dare to cut off a branch or a twig'. He orders them to be 'rooted out and burned'. The stones, which are the object of similar cults in the forests must be 'unearthed completely and cast into a place where they can no longer be venerated'. And the bishop concludes: 'And everybody must be told what a crime idolatry is!'[38]

But the record most strongly reminiscent of Stephen of Bourbon's *exemplum*, because of its hagiographical context, is to be found in the *Life of Saint Martin* written by Sulpicius Severus in about 400. Eight and a half centuries before Stephen of Bourbon described his own experience, Sulpicius Severus told of how the holy Bishop of Tours annihilated a 'superstitious' cult, i.e., one which, in his terms, was a deviation from Christianity or a survival of paganism:[39]

> But to give some indication of all the other 'virtues' he showed during his episcopate, there was a place not far from the town, very near the hermitage that popular belief (*hominium opinio*) took to

be sacred, on the pretext that certain martyrs had been buried there. There was in fact an altar, said to have been set up by previous bishops. But Martin was not prepared to believe in a vague tradition without some kind of confirmation, and at once asked the oldest preachers and clerics to tell him the martyr's name and the date of his passion. When he discovered that tradition could give no coherent or definitive answer on this point, he declared himself extremely worried and uneasy.

For some time, therefore, he refrained from visiting the place, but because of the uncertainty in which he found himself he neither outlawed the cult nor gave the people (*vulgus*) the warrant of his approval, hoping thereby to prevent the superstition growing any stronger. But one day he went to the site, taking some of his brothers with him, and standing above the tomb itself he prayed to the Lord to tell him who was buried there and what his merits were. Then, turning to his left, he saw a loathsome and fierce shadow appear beside him, so he ordered it to declare its name and nature. It declined to give a name but admitted its crime: it had been a brigand, executed for his dreadful crimes, and wrongly venerated by the people (*vulgus*); it had nothing in common with the martyrs, for they dwelt in glory and it in punishment. What was even more remarkable was that those with him heard the voice but were unable to see anything. Then Martin recounted publicly what he had seen and had the altar, which was still there, removed. And thus it was that he delivered the people (*populum*) from the error of this superstition.

Stephen of Bourbon was, of course, familiar with the *Life of Saint Martin*, which was undoubtedly the best-known hagiographical text of the Middle Ages, and quotes several episodes from it in his treatise. The cult denounced by Saint Martin may have entailed the worship of a brigand rather than a dog, but both cases involve the veneration of a false martyr. The steps they take to deal with it are strikingly similar. In both texts doubt as to the identity and name of the saint gives rise to an 'investigation' (though only the Dominican uses the word) which leads to the discovery of the crime. In both cases the churchmen travel to the cult site (*ad locum*). Stephen of Bourbon, who is not a saint, goes there after learning the truth at confession; Saint Martin goes there first and then learns the truth through a miraculous revelation from God. In both cases, the destruction of the cult site takes place in the presence of the people, and in both cases the people are spared, with no punishment incurred by anyone. Finally, the church's victory is in both cases assumed to be definitive.

The widespread influence of the *Life of Saint Martin* can be observed in other medieval documents also. In 743, the *Indiculus superstitionum et paganiarum* denounced, apart from those guilty of 'incantations', and 'sortileges', people who worship 'in dubious places' and who 'make saints for themselves out of ordinary dead persons'.[40] Much later, Sulpicius Severus's testimony is explicitly mentioned in connection with the suppression of a folk cult comparable to that of Saint Guinefort: in August and September 1443, Pierre Soybert, Bishop of Saint Papoul (now the *département* of Aude), had extensive correspondence with the Dominican inquisitor for the province of Toulouse, Hugo Nigri, on the subject of a 'superstitious' and 'idolatrous' curative cult. The cult was celebrated at a place called Les Planhes, where a spring at the foot of a tree that was formerly used as a watering place for pigs was attracting a number of the sick, who prostrated themselves before it and drank the water; they claimed that the holy martyrs Julian and Basilicus were buried there. It had become a place of pilgrimage after a shepherd's cow had miraculously gone down on its knees in front of the spring. . . . But the bishop was adamant: the two saints in question had been martyred at Antioch, and therefore could not possibly be buried at Les Planhes. At best, there might be 'some unmarked grave'. And he went on to quote the example of Saint Martin and the brigand who was improperly venerated as a martyr. In his conclusions he advanced another hypothesis, which is even more reminiscent of Stephen of Bourbon's discovery of a dog–martyr: 'At this spring in Les Planhes there are beasts (*pecora*) which take the place of martyrs. The holy martyrs Julian and Basilicus were martyred at Antioch and not at the place called Les Planhes.' So the cult was prohibited, the spring was filled in, and the pilgrims were threatened with excommunication if there was any recurrence.[41]

Analysis of Stephen of Bourbon's vocabulary and preconceptions, as well as a preliminary survey of his activities, shows his narrative to be part of a long clerical tradition of the suppression of folk culture. But, in order to show in more detail the forces that were reshaping this tradition in the mid thirteenth century, and to show how it was operating in practice, we need now to scrutinise his actions more closely.

3

PREACHING, CONFESSION, INQUISITION

Stephen of Bourbon discovered the 'superstitious' cult of Saint Guinefort while preaching against sortilege and hearing confession. His initial suspicions prompted him to launch an investigation (*inquisivi*) which would seem to have justified making a journey to the scene of the offence ('we travelled to the place'). There he called the people together and preached again, but this time with the specific purpose of condemning the cult in which his listeners had participated. Then he destroyed the cult site and, with the support of the lord of the local estates, forbade any recurrence of the offence.

Stephen of Bourbon was primarily a preacher and a confessor. The two tasks are closely linked in his pastoral practice, in accordance with the mission of the Dominican friars, whose constitution always mentions the preacher's two activities together.[1] Humbert of Romans in his manual of preaching criticises those who preach but refuse to gather the fruits of their preaching in confession.[2]

Conversely, the manuals for Dominican confessors always specify that the preacher must preface confession with at least a short *sermo*, if not a full sermon, to 'arouse the devotion' of those about to make confession, exhorting them 'not to blush to confess their sins' and making much of the sacraments of penance.[3]

It was because he was preaching about sortilege that Stephen of Bourbon was able to make his discovery. It is a type of sermon that comes under the special category of sermons *de diversis*, distinct from the other major classes of medieval sermon, the sermons *de tempore* which comment on the gospel for the day; sermons *de sanctis*, in praise of the saint whose feast day it is; and sermons *ad status*, a genre which developed in the thirteenth century, which were addressed to particular social groups.

Apart from its general theme, we know nothing about the sermon Stephen of Bourbon actually preached. But we can gain some idea of its form and content from looking at other preachers' sermons on the same topic.

The sermons that the Bishop of Paris, Maurice of Sully (1160–96), preached in French against superstition are deservedly famous. But they were preached in special circumstances, at the feast of the Circumcision and the feast of Saint John, to condemn superstitious practices that had developed as part of the celebrations.[4]

There is a Provençal sermon on the Ten Commandments which is undoubtedly closer to the kind of preaching we are trying to define. In it, condemnation of belief in lots, augurs and divination is linked with the First Commandment, which enjoins belief in a single three-person God.[5] Anyone who breaks the First Commandment is guilty of idolatry, the same sin that Bourbon denounces in the cult of Saint Guinefort. In the absence of any sermons which are specifically *de superstitione*, sermons on the Ten Commandments, particularly the First, probably provide the best examples of ecclesiastical condemnation of superstition. The way that the Franciscan, Oliver Maillard, talks of the First Commandment in the famous Lenten sermons he gave at Nantes in 1470 is reminiscent of the very terms that Stephen of Bourbon uses: the preacher is combating superstition and pride simultaneously, because the superstitious worship other gods than God, and the proud worship man himself.[6]

Only one genuine sermon against superstition has survived, and that only indirectly. It is the one delivered by the Bishop of Saint Papoul in September 1443 when he made public his 'conclusions' about the 'idolatrous' cult at Les Planhes. On the feast of Saint Michael, after he had celebrated mass, the bishop 'preached a sermon in the course of which he pronounced these conclusions. He spoke of the superstitions, illusions and errors which, according to the Holy Scriptures, are to be observed at the time of the true and mysterious Antichrist and the foul Satan, and explained the meaning of the passage in Revelation, chapter 16. And there was a great multitude of the people who thronged around and peacefully listened to the word of God.' In fact, it seems unlikely that this sermon would resemble the one given in similar circumstances by Stephen of Bourbon. The bishop's warning (the passage from the Book of Revelation upon which he comments describes God's punishment of 'the men which had the mark of the Beast') has a completely different feeling to it, more appropriate to the fifteenth century and, more particularly, it seems, to that region, for he goes on to say that 'all this should not surprise us, for the kingdom of the devil is close by, in the mountains of the Pyrenees . . . and the arrival of the Antichrist must be heralded by prodigies and misleading signs'.[7]

The last category of sermons, the sermons *ad status*, are therefore more relevant here. In his recommendations to preachers Humbert of Romans warned against the 'poor women' in the villages who were 'much inclined to sortilege, which they use for themselves, for their sons when they are ill, or to protect their animals from wolves'.[8] He states that all women are susceptible to sortilege. But when he describes how it is that one should preach to peasants in general (*ad rusticos*), he makes no mention of it. Preaching manuals are normative in character, and there is basically much more to be learned from the sermons *ad status* themselves, such as the *sermones vulgares* of the secular preacher Jacques de Vitry (1165–1240).

These sermons with their *exempla*, preached in the vernacular but recorded in Latin, are doubly interesting because Stephen of Bourbon had read them and takes a number of *exempla* from them to use in his own collection. He may well have drawn his inspiration to preach against sortilege from some of de Vitry's sermons.

The second of Jacques de Vitry's *Sermones vulgares*, intended for 'widows and chaste women', praises the virtues of penitence, which provides a defence against the trickeries of sorcerers (*malefici*) and soothsayers. Eight *exempla* are then cited, each following on from the one before and, in fact, comprise the bulk of the sermon. They all provide evidence of the treachery of demons and witches (*malefici mulieres*), of the deceitful old woman (*vetula fallax*), or the sacrilegious old woman who casts lots (*vetula sacrilega et sortilega*). A short commentary, interspersed with quotations from 'authorities' (basically Saint Paul and Saint Augustine) provides the transition from one *exemplum* to the next. A more substantial conclusion reminds the audience how 'women who cast lots' offend against the sacraments of the church 'from the cradle to the grave' (*a principio autem nativitatis usque ad senectutem et mortem*). Thus the preacher adjures mothers to bring up their sons and daughters to fear sortilege.[9] There is every reason to believe that Bourbon's sermon would have been similar to this.

After preaching, he heard people's confessions and thereby learnt what superstitions they were guilty of. In fact, questions about superstition were a normal part of confessional interrogation.

Examination for superstitious beliefs was considered a crucial aspect of the penitential practices of the early Middle Ages, and this continued to be the case until the twelfth century. This vigilance was originally justified by the need to root out paganism, and then by the need to convert the 'barbarians' who were living within Western Christendom. Which is why penitentials – the catalogues of offences and tarifs of punishment – provide such ample documentation on the subject of superstitions.

This is particularly the case with the *Decretum* and *Corrector sive medicus* which Bishop Burchard of Worms wrote shortly after the year 1000,[10] and with Alan of Lille's *Liber penitentialis*, written in the twelfth century.[11]

But from the twelfth century a new type of confession develops which is individual, based on the special relationship between confessor and sinner, and designed to take account of the specific circumstances in which each sin was committed, and of the sinner's *intention* in particular. The Lateran Council's canon *Omnis utriusque sexus* of 1215 decreed that every Christian had to attend confession at least once a year, at Easter, and the mendicant orders did much to ensure that this was enforced during the thirteenth century. In order to administer the sacrament of penance in its new form confessors needed to have some kind of reference grid of sins to help them examine sinners, and this is the context in which the success of the '*Summas* of Vices and Virtues', which became necessary complements to the confessor's manuals, should be seen. Even before the Lateran Council, these manuals tended to be organised around the Seven Vices, so that when the confessor had gone through the list of all the Vices, he and the penitent could part, knowing that no sin had been committed.

Superstitions had therefore to be linked with one of the Seven Vices, and Stephen of Bourbon, writing in about 1255–61, chose *Superbia*, Pride. This choice should perhaps be seen as a sign that the process of integrating superstition into the new penitential system had been successfully completed. Half a century earlier, in Thomas of Cobham's manual of confession, sortilege had not really found its place among the Vices. The author links it rather tenuously to murder, by way of malefic poisoning, which is a consequence of *Ira*, Anger. This puts sortilege just before *Avaritia*, which is clearly a provisional placing, and one that implies a search for a classificatory system, but it also underlines the significance of sortilege, which is put on an equal footing with the Seven Vices.[12]

Stephen of Bourbon shows no hesitation, just a few years later, in linking superstitions to *Superbia*. Therefore, when he heard confession from the local peasants, he must have examined them on all the sins deriving from the Vice of Pride. And, coming to superstition, he discovered the existence of the cult of Saint Guinefort.

Having heard during confession the admissions his preaching had aroused, Stephen of Bourbon made his investigation (*inquisivi*). The word is important because it alludes to the inquisitorial procedure which developed in the first half of the thirteenth century, and to the office of inquisition with which Stephen of Bourbon had been charged since 1235. It is a procedure in which the judge himself conducts the investigation, provoking denunciations and admissions, not waiting passively for offenders to be brought to him, as in accusatory proceedings. Did Stephen of Bourbon in fact behave as an inquisitor during this affair?

When he describes his activities against heretics, he uses the same word: 'When I was making investigations against the heretics. . .' ('cum ego inquirerem de hereticis'), he says frequently, before going on to specify whether or not he found something or somebody suspicious. Only twice, in fifteen cases, does he say that he was proceeding 'by apostolic mandate' or 'in the office of inquisition'.

Nor does he usually make any distinction between his activities as an inquisitor and his activities as a preacher and confessor: 'as I have found in numerous inquisitions and confessions. . .', 'as I was preaching against the Albigensian heretics. . .'.[13] His approach is many-sided, as one can see in the case of the cult of Saint Guinefort, where the three activities of preaching, confession and inquisition are closely connected and all play their part in the uncovering of deviance – sometimes heresy, but in this case superstition.

This must clearly have been the Pope's intention when he bestowed the office of inquisition upon the mendicant orders, in that they specialised in preaching and in the new confession. One of the reasons for the promulgation, in 1215, of the canon *Omnis utriusque sexus* on the new confession may have been the desire for a more efficacious means of discovering heretics.[14] The inquisitor had to be a preacher too: when Humbert of Romans listed all the possible types of sermon for the Dominicans, he included instructions on how to preach 'at a formal inquisition', 'at an inquisition after the discovery of a crime', 'at the end of an inquisition after the discovery of a crime', 'at the inquisition of heretics', and 'at the condemnation of heretics'.[15]

Sermons in fact framed the inquisitorial proceedings. They opened with a sermon which provided a few moments' grace for spontaneous admissions, and concluded with the *sermo generalis*, which was delivered at a public session where all the *people* were called together, with the representatives of the secular power, to whom the condemned were ultimately delivered.[16] This minutely ordered procedure did not assume its final shape until the second half of the fourteenth century, when it was set out by the Catalan Dominican inquisitor, Nicolau Eymerich, in his *Directorium inquisitorium* (*c*. 1376). But Stephen of Bourbon probably followed much the same procedure in the present case: the concluding sermon is a response to the initial one and denounces the offence in front of the assembled people (*populus*), while the support of the secular power is sought to preempt any actual recurrence.

The word *populus*, in the idiom of the church, meant the Christian community of a diocese or parish. When the inquisitors use the word, 'the people called together' for the formal sermon often meant the whole population of a town. But most of Stephen of Bourbon's work was in rural parishes, whose composition seemed very simple to him, with the curé (*sacerdos*) at the head, followed (more or less closely) by his parishioners (*parochiani*).[17]

In the present case, the word *populus* is inseparable from the word *terra*, and means the people of an estate belonging to a lord. Bourbon uses the word 'estate' (*terre*) elsewhere in the collection,[18] but nowhere else is the meaning as clear as it is here, where it refers to the *dominium* of a lord; the 'people of the estate' are thus the individuals under his power.[19] It is to their lord that Stephen of Bourbon makes his appeal, as is the prerogative of his status as inqusititor.[20]

Inquisitors did not concern themselves with secular punishment. In their campaign against heresy they tried cases, passed judgement and, when appropriate, imposed spiritual penances such as pilgrimages. They never pronounced the death penalty themselves, but delivered convicted offenders into the care of the secular authorities. At the request of an inquisitor, an offender's possessions were confiscated by the civil authorities, declared public property and sold at auction. Somebody who had been convicted but whose life had been spared could not reclaim his possessions until he had completely discharged his penance.[21] This is obviously the meaning of the edict that was promulgated at Stephen of Bourbon's request, which confirms that he did indeed act as an inquisitor from start to finish.

The lord who gave the inquisitor his support still has to be identified. Stephen of Bourbon discovered the location of the cult site of Saint Guinefort upon the 'estate of the lord of Villars', and it was the 'lords of the estate' whom he asked to make an edict.

There are in fact a number of charters testifying to the powers of the lords of Villars in this region.[22] Two allied families succeeded one another to the head of this seigneury during the Middle Ages. One, first recorded in 1030, became famous in the mid twelfth century through Stephen II of Villars, who bore the title of 'lord' (*sire; dominus*). Having no son ('cum non habebat prolem sive heredem') he gave a part of his possessions to the Abbey of Saint Sulpice when he left to go on a crusade in 1145. When he returned in 1148 he built (between 1163 and 1170) the Cistercian Abbey of Chassagne, 'daughter' of the one at Saint Sulpice, on the land he had bequeathed. In 1186 he entered the monastery of Ile-Barbe.

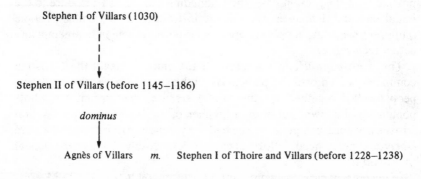

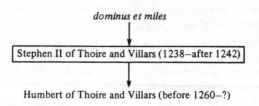

Table 1 *Succession of the lords of Villars*

Sometime before 1228 his daughter Agnès married Stephen of Thoire, 'lord and knight' (*dominus et miles*), who succeeded his stepfather to the title of 'lord of Thoire and Villars'. He was succeeded in 1238 by their son, Stephen of Thoire and Villars, who not long after went to Cremona to pay homage to the Emperor for all his fiefs of the Empire, on the East of the Saône. He is probably the lord to whom Stephen of Bourbon made his appeal. Stephen was succeeded by his son, Humbert of Thoire and Villars, who in 1260 released the men of the Abbey of Chassagne from the rent they were paying 'for his estate of Villars' ('pro terra sua de Villars').

It is more difficult to identify the lands of the lords of Villars in the immediate vicinity of Neuville-les-Dames and along the Chalaronne. Other families, as well as ecclesiastical foundations, had rights and possessions in the region: the lords of Beaujeu (Guichard, then Humbert), were receiving the homage of Châtillon-sur-Chalaronne and had rights over Sandrans. Romans, on the other hand, although very close, was held in fief from the lords of Bâgé by Ulrich of Varax.

In using his position as inquisitor to suppress the cult of Saint Guinefort, Stephen of Bourbon was proceeding against superstition rather than heresy, which was his usual target. Does this mean that he was overstepping his normal powers? The question is all the more pertinent if one bears in mind that, once the inquisitor had begun to preach 'against sortilege', he was clearly intending to hunt out superstitions. He did not discover them in the course of an inquisition against heretics.

The tribunal of the Inquisition was, admittedly, set up to combat all possible deviations in matters of faith, but to begin with its only explicit concern was with heresy. The campaign against superstition, particularly against witchcraft, was a gradual extension of the inquisitor's mission. The Council of Valence in 1248 still set 'witches and sacrileges' under the ordinary jurisdiction of bishops, not the Inquisition, and moreover kept them distinct from heretics.[23] But, in reply to questions from the Franciscans and Dominicans working in Italy, Pope Alexander IV made two replies, on 13 December 1258 and on 10 January 1260 respectively, which indicate that a distinct change had occurred. They were anxious to know 'if it is within the scope of inquisitors of heresy to recognise cases of divination and sortilege that are reported to them, and to punish those who take part in them'. The Pope replied that matters of faith (*negotium fidei*) must take precedence, and that, consequently, the inquisitors should not treat cases of divination and sortilege 'unless they obviously savour of heresy' (*nisi manifeste saperent haeresim*). Other cases should continue to be the responsibility of the episcopal courts.[24] The same distinction occurs in Alexander IV's bull *Quod super nonnullis*. The next development was in 1270, when the first inquisitor's manual devoted to superstitions appeared, the *Summa de officio inquisitionis*, which would seem to have originated in the Bishop of Marseilles's entourage, and which provides appropriate questions to ask when trying 'augurs and idolaters' (*Forma et modus interrogandi augures et ydolatras*).[25] Do they worship demons? Do they make invocations to demons or plants, birds or other creatures, etc.? But they are never actually described as 'heretics'.

The next development is marked by Bernard Gui's *Inquisitor's Manual*. He was inquisitor at Toulouse from about 1307 to 1323.[26] The vocabulary is now settled; the 'casters of lots, soothsayers, and invokers of demons' are denounced (*De sortilegis et divinis et invocatoribus demonum*). It echoes the rigid formula of the papal bulls, and thereafter there are few changes. Even if the correct distinction between 'sortilege' and 'divination' continued to be the subject of debate in the fourteenth century, the inflexibility of the official formula settled the terminological uncertainty of half a century earlier. And additionally, although inquisitors were particularly eager to uncover cases having 'the savour of heresy', they now had to concern themselves with all the other cases too; a form of words to be used in recantations is aimed 'primarily at cases which have the savour of heresy', but seems not to have been restricted to these alone. Thus, the whole vocabulary of inquisitorial proceedings against heresy comes to be applied to 'sortilege, divination and invocation of demons': these are described as 'various and multiform plagues and delusions occurring in different estates and different regions', in exactly the same way as the Cathar and Waldensian heresies.

There were yet further developments, however. For the increasing sophistication of both inquisitorial practice and demonological theory led, especially after 1480, to wholesale persecution of witches. But it is only necessary to look at the first stages in this process in order to provide a more accurate context for Stephen of Bourbon's actions in the Saint Guinefort affair.

Although he was one of the first inquisitors, Stephen of Bourbon used the inquisitorial procedure against superstition some twenty years before the Pope had officially instructed inquisitors to try superstitions which had the 'savour of heresy'. Stephen of Bourbon's initiative, and the questions that the Italian inquisitors put to Pope Alexander IV, are confirmation that the pontifical instructions merely ratified and encouraged a practice that inquisitors were already using in the field.

The sentences pronounced by the inquisitors at the end of the proceedings also changed as the system evolved. Compared with the punishments meted out to heretics in the same period, Stephen of Bourbon's clemency is remarkable. Elsewhere in the treatise he speaks quite coolly of the torture of 'an old Manichaean woman' from Champagne, and of dozens of heretics from Mont-Aimé.[27] The clemency shown to the women who made the pilgrimage to the tomb of Saint Guinefort, and, more particularly, to the *vetula* who taught them the rite, is very different from the severity of the punishments dealt out to witches in the fiteenth century, as enumerated in the *Malleus maleficarum* in 1486.[28] There is not a single reference to physical punishment in those *exempla* in which Stephen of Bourbon discusses superstitions. He even exonerated a woman from Forez accused of witchcraft, who had been brought before him by a curé at the request of his parishioners.[29]

The first reason for such clemency has already been given: in Stephen of Bourbon's time there was still very little common ground between heresy and witchcraft. Both stemmed from *Superbia*, Pride. But whereas he believed heresy to be the domain of dogmatic error (*error*) consciously held and rationally defended, superstition was a matter of diabolic trickery (*ludificatio*), in which man is more victim than participant. The 'sophisms' of the heretics in their 'sects', preaching subversion against the church, had to be met with the 'demonstration' of the articles of the faith, the 'reasons' and 'disputations'. If the heretics persisted, moreover, they would have to be burned. But it was only necessary to unmask the meddling of the devil that underlay the illusions of a superstitious old woman for that 'simple soul' to be brought back to the right path.[30]

Heresy and witchcraft remain largely separate in Stephen of Bourbon's mind, then, because he thinks of each as having a specific nature, and entailing particular dangers. But this difference has a chronological aspect too, for so long as inquisitors were dealing with heretics, superstition did not seem to warrant the same severity. This attitude was still in evidence at the beginning of the fourteenth century, when Jacques Fournier, Bishop of Pamiers, was hunting down the last Cathar *parfaits** in the valleys of Upper Ariège, but ignoring peasant supersititions, even though they were far more discrepant with contemporary catholic orthodoxy.[31] Once heresy had been eradicated, the inquisitors could turn their attention to witches. In fact, that is precisely what the inquisitor Hugo Nigri said to the Bishop of Saint Papoul on 4 September 1443, as an excuse for not having replied earlier to the Bishop's letter of 14 August regarding the superstitious cult at Les Planhes. Being absorbed in a delicate question of heresy, the inquisitor had felt himself obliged 'to neglect all other matters'.

Another reason for Stephen of Bourbon's clemency was the 'simplicity' of the peasants whose superstitious cult he destroyed. A few years earlier the inquisitor Robert le Bougre had been convicted of abusing his inquisitorial powers, and had been criticised for launching the same persecution against truly 'wicked' heretics and people who were adjudged merely 'innocent and simple'.[32] Stephen of Bourbon did not make that sort

---

*The Cathars (Albigensians) were divided into ordinary believers and a pure, baptised élite, the *parfaits*, who from the moment of their initiation abstained from meat and women and had the power to bless bread and believers. *Tr.*

of mistake, for simple peasants (*rustici*) did not in his view merit the same treatment as dangerous heretics.

His attitude to *rusticitas* was admittedly an ambiguous one. It may be compared with *ignobilitas* (loss of nobility) and had long been marked with the stigma of servitude (while *nobilitas*, says Stephen of Bourbon, is characterised by the state of liberty [*liberalitas*]); it naturally drove people to crime, for *rusticitas*, the author reminds us, means 'stealing' (*auferre*), 'committing crimes' (*malefacere*), 'pillaging' ('rusticitas est furari vel rapere').[33] Yet rusticity had positive qualities too, and, as a member of a mendicant order, Stephen of Bourbon is aware that the peasants are poor, denied power, knowledge and wealth, and therefore secure from the temptations they bring. The simplicity of their lives, their customs and their thoughts is the natural form of the virtue of humility. Witness the mother of Bishop Maurice of Sully, a 'poor, rustic, uneducated little woman, who never thought of self-adornment'.[34] But the day she began to dress up and paint her face her saintly son no longer recognised her. The simplicity of the *rustici* makes them very vulnerable to temptation. They are quick to be taken in, too, by the tricks of rogues and scoundrels (*truffatores*).[35] And, above all, they are ideal victims for the devil's illusions. Their temptations correspond to the frustration of their lives and the insecure image of their own desires.[36] But it is not too grave a thing for them to fall. Indeed, unlike the heretic who 'takes refuge in sophisms' when he is interrogated, the simple man (*homo simplex et planus*) knows nothing of the subtleties of argument. The inquisitor's task is therefore easier, for 'either he gives the right answer or the wrong one. If he gives the wrong one he receives correction and instruction'.[37] This is exactly what Stephen of Bourbon did with the peasants who venerated Saint Guinefort.

The majority of these peasants were women and were, as such, even more susceptible to the advances of the devil. Stephen of Bourbon was, in this respect, simply a creature of his own time. Only noble women deserved flattering portraits.[38] Yet distrust and scorn did not prevent Stephen of Bourbon from showing a degree of indulgence. Even in the case of old women (*vetule*) who were in league with the devil, Stephen of Bourbon fulminated and condemned but never used violence. He denounced the work of the devil, but he did not seek to have the victims burned. Even when they prophesied the future and cast lots (*divinatrix, sortilega*), he saw them first and foremost as simple souls led astray by the devil.[39] There was even one *vetula* – who, it is true, did not cast lots – who won Stephen of Bourbon's approval, for every day, drenched in tears, she would recite the Paternoster, the Ave, and the Credo until a dove appeared to console her. Moved by her piety, the bishop wanted her to learn the Psalter as well, whereupon she lost the gift of tears and the dove did not reappear. Everything returned to normal when she reverted to her old prayers, which thus came to be seen as the ideal and sufficient prayers for simple lay people in the thirteenth century.[40] There was one *vetula*, on the other hand, who was burned, but she, as we have seen, was clearly a heretic. In between these two extremes, the great mass of *vetule* cast lots, interpret omens, foretell the future, and sometimes invoke demons. The author denounces them vigorously, but his condemnations have a touch of irony about them also. The diminutive *vetule* (these little old ladies!) sets the tone. And thus the *vetula*, in the thirteenth century, is still treated mercifully. In the fifteenth century, on the other hand, the *malefica* is burned without hesitation, for she can be convicted of harming her neighbours – threatening their lives, their sexual potency or the health of their cattle – with the aid of the devil. Whereas, around 1250, the *vetula* in the *exemplum* simply invoked demons to save the lives of young children.

Admittedly, Stephen of Bourbon did not see it in these terms. He accused the women of infanticide, yet without threatening them with severe punishment. Here too his indulgence may seem surprising. Since the early Middle Ages the church had constantly denounced infanticide, which it originally looked upon as a sin, punishable by canon law alone. From the thirteenth century onwards infanticide was increasingly seen as a crime, to be investigated and tried by the lay judges, and entailing the possibility of a death sentence where intent could be proved, or for second offenders.[41] The most common infanticidal practices in this period are the abandonment or exposure of children, suffocation of new-born babies in their parents' bed, and various simulated accidents (when a child is left to play near a vat of boiling water, there is a likelihood of his falling in . . .). Stephen of Bourbon probably did not regard this cult as ritual infanticide, which would have forced him to adopt far more severe measures, but saw it merely in the light of the danger to children's lives that it represented. Hence, again, his remarkable clemency. But it also raises the full complexity of the question of the cult's real function: how was it that the cult came to be connected, beyond any doubt, with the then crucial matter of infanticide, when its central purpose was not to kill children but to save their lives?

PART 2

The legend and the rite

4

THE LEGEND

Although the document under study is a product of learned culture and represssion, it nonetheless provides quite vivid and precise information about folk culture, which is rarely the case with medieval documents.

In the course of describing his own activities, Stephen of Bourbon also set down what the peasants told him about their beliefs and their customs. There is no doubt, of course, that putting other people's words into writing, making a Latin version of a vernacular narrative, does some violence to the original folk culture. But that is no reason to reject the evidence and abandon the investigation. An *exemplum* is a short narrative, and it is unlikely that Stephen of Bourbon recorded all that he was told. He had to make a synthesis of all the information he gathered during confession, but he does not seem to have distorted it. The internal coherence of the narrative as a whole seems, on the contrary, to confirm the trustworthiness of the evidence.

The evidence about folk culture that Stephen of Bourbon provides can be divided into two parts: a narrative in the past tense about the origins of the cult site, and a description of the healing rite itself.

These two parts will each be subjected to the same type of analysis: in each case this will consist of a formal analysis, examining the narrative or ritual sequences and their connections, and a semantic analysis of the essential elements of the narrative. I shall then examine the hagiographic literature regarding Saint Guinefort, and I shall try to trace the history of the cult. Only then shall I try to interpret the document in historical terms, surveying it as a whole, and in a way that cannot be done in these preliminary analyses.[1]

Neither the peasants whose confession Stephen of Bourbon heard, nor the inquisitor himself, had any doubts about the authenticity of the narrative of the dog's death, and this certainty informed both the peasants' belief and the inquisitor's decision to suppress it. But we know that the same story is to be found in plenty of other places and periods too. It elaborates a 'motif' that is well known in oral literature, indexed in the international classification under numbers B524ff.[2]

I would therefore define this narrative as a legend both in the usual sense of the term, in that the wealth of different versions indicates that it is not a 'true story', and also in the technical sense of a particular narrative genre. If we employ the formal criteria that adherents of the traditional classification of narrative genres use, this version of the story of the faithful dog can in fact be defined as a legend (*la légende, die Sage*), rather than as a hagiographic legend (*la légende hagiographique, die Legende*), or those of a folktale (*le conte, das Märchen*); it adopts its historical perspective ('the folktale is basically poetic, the legend basically historical', writes Hermann Bausinger), it also has the legend's concrete setting, the theme of the family, and a narrative which ends with the hero's death (whereas the folktale often ends before the hero dies). The absence of Christian motifs, or their fragmentary presence, is also characteristic of the *Sage* rather than the *Legende*. It is also worth noting that the titles of 'saint' and 'martyr', and even the name 'Guinefort', are not given to the greyhound in the legend itself, but either before or after it, in the text of the *exemplum*.[3] Adherents of formal systems of classification have warned, however, against the dangers of using the categories they propose in too rigid a manner. Bausinger, in particular, lays less stress on the separate genres than on the areas of overlap (*Übergangslandschaft*) which link them. The document itself also forewarns us against another temptation, namely that when scholars study these accounts in versions abstracted from their context and inserted into 'collections of folktales and legends', they all too often tend to forget the people whose words these are, and the social and historical conditions in which they were spoken.

The corpus of narratives

The narrative is recorded in a very similar form in the Sanskrit literature of India in the sixth century B.C. It forms part of the *Pañchatantra*, a treatise on the education of princes. It features in the fifth and final part of this treatise, which teaches the prince to guard against hasty action and rash behaviour.[4] A summary of this should suffice.

A son had just been born to a brahman and his wife. On the same day their female mongoose gave birth to a baby, which the brahman's wife raised as her own. One day the brahmanee had to go out and entrusted the child to the brahman. But he went out in his turn, leaving the child alone with the mongoose. Shortly afterwards a black snake emerged from a hole and was about to attack the child when the mongoose saved him by killing the snake. When the mother returned she saw the mongoose's bloodstained jaws, thought it had eaten her child, and killed it. But when she went into the room she found the child safe and sound, and the body of the snake in pieces. She realised her mistake, and was very much distressed. When the brahman returned she upbraided him for going out despite what she had said, and held him responsible for the death of their mongoose 'son'.

Independently of the Indian narrative, which is still a part of Indian oral tradition, another, quite different version was recorded by Pausanias in

Greece, about A.D. 160–80. This one was an 'aetiological' legend of a city, Amphicleia in Phocis,[5] whose inhabitants spoke as follows:

> A certain chief, suspecting that enemies were plotting against his baby son, put the child in a vessel, and hid him in that part of the land where he knew there would be most security. Now a wolf attacked the child, but a serpent coiled itself round the vessel, and kept up a strict watch. When the child's father came, supposing that the serpent had purposed to attack the child, he threw his javelin, which killed the serpent and his son as well. But being informed by the shepherds that he had killed the benefactor and protector of his child, he made one common pyre for both the serpent and his son. Now they say that even today the place resembles a burning pyre, maintaining that after this serpent the City was called Ophiteia.

The Greek version is clearly quite different from the Indian one, for in it the snake is the child's protector and not the aggressor; the child is killed, but by his father, etc. The Greek version seems quite independent of the long series of oriental works that stem from the *Pañchatantra*.

The *Pañchatantra* was in fact very popular in the East. Shortly before A.D. 570 a Sassanian prince had it translated into Pahlavi. After the Arab invasion of 652, that same translation, which is now lost, was translated into Arabic by order of the Caliph al-Mansur in the eighth century. This Arabic version was made by Ibn al-Muqaffa', and was given the title *The Book of Kalila and Dimna*. A Greek translation was made in the late eleventh century, perhaps by a certain Simeon, son of Seth. It was translated into Hebrew in the mid thirteenth century by Rabbi Joël as the *Mishle Sendabat*. It was this last work which was translated into Latin between 1263 and 1278 by a converted Jew, John of Capua, under the title of *Directorium humanae vitae.*[6]

The first Latin translation of this story does not therefore appear in the West until several years after Stephen of Bourbon's death. Which means that the peasant version of *c.* 1250 cannot be directly related to the corpus of narratives whose tradition I have just traced.

The peasant legend of 1250 is not the earliest recorded version in Latin Christian culture. There is a version in Old French, dated *c.* 1155, in the earliest known version of the *Roman des sept sages*. The *Dolopathos*, a Latin treatise written by the Lorraine Cistercian, John of Haute Seille, in about 1184, also predates the *exemplum*, and *a fortiori* John of Capua's translation. This work was translated into French in the thirteenth century by someone called Herbert.

These two treatises, the *Roman des sept sages* and the *Dolopathos*, are similar in both conception and execution, and also resemble those works belonging to the long tradition deriving from the *Pañchatantra*. Both recount the adventures of a young prince who is raised away from home by a tutor, following the death of his mother, and is then sent for by his father when he remarries. But, before he leaves, his master advises him to feign dumbness from the moment he arrives at court. Confident of his silence, his stepmother tries to seduce him, but, failing in this aim, she accuses the young man of trying to rape her. The king wants to have his son put to death, but seven wise men dissuade him by telling one or two stories each, in order to illustrate the harmful consequences of hasty action. One of the stories is that of the faithful dog. The king ends by pardoning his son, whose innocence is discovered at the end of the book.

There is clearly some connection between these two treatises and the oriental treatises on education. But the channels through which they were transmitted are not known to us. It seems likely, however, that Simeon-Seth's Greek translation at the end of the eleventh century provided the necessary link. Yet, while the oriental influence is visible in the general composition of these works, and in the subject matter of some of the narratives that they contain, oriental precedents cannot be found for all of the narratives: this is particularly the case with the *Dolopathos*, for which John of Haute-Seille also collected original narratives locally.

How then did the peasant legend recorded in the mid thirteenth century by Stephen of Bourbon first arise? There are two possible hypotheses. First, that the legend is a popularised version of the narratives of Western learned culture, and thus indirectly linked with the oriental narratives whose traditions we have traced. This is, *a priori*, the least attractive option, for it is diffusionist, and involves a facile recourse to explanation in terms of 'influence' (unmasked as long ago as 1893 by Joseph Bédier,[7] but all too often invoked, even nowadays). Moreover, we have no knowledge of the conditions under which this popularisation of a learned narrative would have occurred, whether it would have involved particular clerics as intermediaries, or the local aristocracy.

There are, nevertheless, arguments in favour of this hypothesis. There were, for instance, sufficient exchanges between learned and folk culture, and between aristocracy and peasantry, in the twelfth and thirteenth centuries, to make such popularisation possible. It is also worth bearing in mind the close relationship between this legend and the *Roman des sept sages*. It contrasts quite strikingly, on the other hand, with the independent versions presented in the *Pañchatantra* and by Pausanias, which, although admittedly coming from very different places and times, are divergent in the manner outlined above.

Finally, there have been real advances in recent years in the study of the diffusion of the motifs of oral traditions in relation to African folktales in particular.[8]

In principle, I would favour the second hypothesis, so long as there is some basis for it. According to this hypothesis, the peasant legend of the faithful greyhound would owe nothing at all to external influences. It would be a part of the oral tradition of the local peasantry, and would stem from an ancient Indo-European source. Membership of a common Indo-European community would then account for the same story being found in India as well as in France and in Greece. Yet the anteriority of the two learned versions, in the *Roman des sept sages* and the *Dolopathos*, conflicts with this hypothesis, as does, yet more strongly, the close relationship between these texts and the peasant legend.

We can decide between these two hyptheses only by examining the legend and its parallel versions very thoroughly.

A preliminary survey reveals a number of narratives, from various places and times, that parallel the one with which we began. It is already clear that no interpretation of the document, and in particular of the part that the legend of the faithful dog plays in it, can possibly be advanced until we know the narrative group to which it belongs, and the place it has within it.

Owing to the formal differences between the narratives, which I shall now analyse, the versions that parallel the reference-narrative (N1) have been arranged in three equally important groups.

First Group

All but one of the nine narratives in this group belong to versions of the *Roman des sept sages* written between the twelfth and fourteenth centuries. These versions are listed here in the order in which they were classified by Gaston Paris,[9] and not in chronological order:

N2: narrative of the dog in *Les sept sages de Rome*, rhymed version in French, thirteenth century. G. Paris: version D.[10]

N3: narrative of the dog in *Historia septem sapientium*, Latin MS of 1342. G. Paris: version H.[11]

N4: narrative of the dog in *L'Ystoire des sept sages*. A French adaptation of the previous work.[12]

N5: narrative of the dog in the Latin version known as *Versio italica*, fourteenth century. G. Paris: version I.[13]

N6: narrative of the dog in *Li Romans des sept sages*, in French verse, *c.* 1155. G. Paris: version K.[14]

N7: narrative of the dog in the *Roman des sept sages*, in French prose, thirteenth to fourteenth century. G. Paris: version L.[15]

N8: narrative of the dog in the *Liber de septem sapientibus*, mid thirteenth century, lost but transmitted in an abridged form by Jean Gobi, *Scala celi, c.* 1330, in Latin. G.Paris: version S.[16]

Another version can perhaps be included in this group, although it does not belong to the *Roman des sept sages* series:

N9: narrative of the dog in the Anglo-Latin version of the *Gesta Romanorum*, a collection of moralised *exempla* in Latin, from the fourteenth century.[17]

Second group

N10: narrative of the dog in John of Haute-Seille, *Dolopathos sive de rege et septem sapientibus*, in Latin, c. 1184–1212.[18]

N11: narrative of the dog in *Li Romans de Dolopathos*, French adaptation of the preceding work by Herbert, c. 1223.[19]

The chief originality of these two versions is that they preface the narrative of the death of the dog with a narrative about the knight and his family. Briefly, it is as follows:

A 'youth' (*juvenis*) of noble lineage is anxious to further his reputation by his exploits and his largesse, and to gather a plentiful retinue of companions about him. But when he comes into his inheritance he is unable to settle down and he continues his spendthrift life. His friends warn him to be more prudent but he spurns their advice and accuses them of 'envy'. Sure enough, he is soon destitute. Deeply ashamed and repentant, but 'too late', he leaves the district, accompanied only by his wife, his new-born son, his horse, his hawk and his hound.

After many wanderings he comes at last one evening to a city, where one of the citizens offers him lodging in a house some distance away from the others, which has been uninhabited for years. The knight refuses to work with his hands, or to beg. But each day he goes hunting with his three beasts, and brings home game to feed his family.

One evening he comes back empty-handed. He decides to go out the next day without his dog, which he ties up inside the house. While he is away his wife, afraid that the child will die of hunger, goes to ask a noble lady living nearby for some food. The sequel is the same as the narrative in Stephen of Bourbon's *exemplum*.

Third group

N12: narrative of someone who killed his dog, by Johannes Pauli, *Schimpf und Ernst*, in German, c. 1520.[20]

This narrative is classified separately because it is of slightly later date than the others, and because the knight is the sole protagonist. There is no nurse, and the wife only appears at the end of the narrative to give her husband, the hound's murderer, permission to enter a monastery.

An engraving from the Strasbourg edition of 1535 should be compared with this narrative; it depicts the actual moment when the knight kills his dog. This engraving will be considered on its own account, and not simply as an illustration of the text (Illustration 1).

In all, the corpus comprises twelve narratives and an iconographic document. Each is a product of Western European civilisation between the middle of the twelfth and the beginning of the sixteenth century. Other versions have been omitted, in order to maintain the homogeneity of the corpus.

In my analysis and explication I shall disregard the oriental versions (*Pañchatantra*, Pausanias etc.), since they belong to different cultural backgrounds. Even John of Capua's translation is excluded from the corpus, because it has too strong an oriental stamp for it to be put on the same footing as the other stories. For example, the child's father is a hermit – a transformation of the 'pious Mohameddan' of the *Book of Kalila and Dimna*, who in turn replaced the brahman of the *Pañchatantra* – rather than a knight, as in all the versions of the corpus.[21]. And not just this one character but the whole framework of the narrative is different. The differences do not of course preclude a formal comparison between this narrative and the versions in the corpus, but content analysis cannot, I believe, be divorced from structural analysis, and this narrative clearly requires a quite different interpretation from that proposed for the versions retained here.

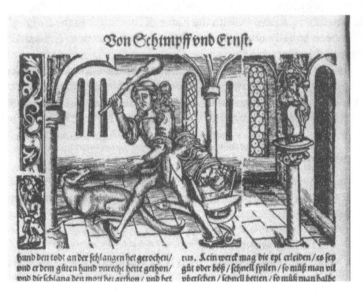

1 The knight kills his dog with a club. Johannes Pauli, *Schimpf und Ernst*. Strasbourg, B. Greininger, 1535, fol. XLVIv (photograph courtesy of the Bibliothèque Nationale, Paris).

Two recent versions of the same narrative have been likewise excluded. One is the Welsh legend of Llywelyn and his hound Gelert. The earliest written account dates only from 1800, when W. R. Spencer wrote a poem about it.[22] But in fact the legend is certainly far older, or so one would suppose from looking at an illustration in the chronicle of John Rous (1483–4), dedicated to the Earls of Warwick, which represents Richard III between his wife and the Prince of Wales. At the latter's feet is a crest, surmounting the Welsh arms, and depicting a greyhound lying in a cradle[23] (Illustration 2). This heraldic detail is not known to occur anywhere else, and must certainly have something to do with the legend that concerns us here. But unfortunately we have no contemporary and local version of the legend.

I shall also disregard the legend of the holy dog Ganelon, recorded in 1713, which is closest, in thematic terms, to the reference-narrative. Indeed this faithful dog, too, was 'canonised' by peasants and the site of his martyrdom became the focus of a healing cult.[24] But it is not because this narrative is recorded at a substantially later date than the others that it is not being included, although it would be awkward to break the chronological unity of the corpus. The main reason is that nothing is known about the legend, neither the conditions in which it was collected, nor the local traditions with which it might ultimately be linked (according to the text, the events took place 'in the Auvergne'). My researches into the dog's name and its possible relationship with the name of the traitor in the *Song of Roland* have been equally unproductive.[25] Given this situation, it seemed wiser to discard this narrative.[26]

Having explained the rules and limitations according to which the corpus was assembled, we can now proceed to a comparative analysis of the various versions. However, the reference-narrative will continue to be the most important one, since it is associated with the cult of Saint Guinefort.

Formal analysis

In my formal analysis of the different versions contained within the corpus, I shall consider in turn, place and time, actors and actions, and the logic of the narrative.

1. Place and time

In the reference-narrative (N1), the action takes place in a castle, which is not described; we simply learn, and fairly late, that it has a door, and beside this door, a well. Nor are we told much about the castle's surroundings, and no description of the interior is given. There is simply an 'outside' – into which people 'go out' – and an 'inside' that the protagonists of the story enter. On the other hand, the castle is carefully situated within the forms of legal 'space' that were then current in that region; this space is defined by a threefold reference to the ecclesiastical district (diocese of Lyons), the monastic network (the convent at Neuville) and lay jurisdiction (on the estate of the lord of Villars).

The action takes place in an indefinite past ('fuit quoddam castro' . . .), and there is nothing to indicate the time of year.

At the end of the narrative, an undeclared amount of time after the murder of the greyhound, the setting alters. The castle has been destroyed and the estate reduced to the condition of a 'desert'.

In the other narratives, the setting is noticeably different, with respect to both space and time. Three versions of the *Roman des sept sages*, however, closely resemble the legend in this respect: in N3 and N4 the action takes place in a knight's castle, in fact in the great hall, or *aula*: the serpent comes out of a hole in the wall. In N8, it is a farmhouse outside the town, with meadows and a spring, entirely surrounded with 'very old, ruined walls', out of which the serpent comes.

All the other versions of the *Roman des sept sages* explictly place the action in an urban setting, in Rome. The knight's home is a town house or a castle close by the town walls, and its interior is clearly described: the room, the cradle, a kneading trough, another bed, the door (which the nurses shut behind them), the window (through which the snake enters) (N2 and N6). In N7 the house gives on to a courtyard. Nearby is the wall of the 'great and ancient' (N2) town, riddled with holes. It is crenellated and the town gate has a drawbridge. Only in N5 does the whole narrative take place within the town (the knight and his family have gone to the Roman games in the market square, 'ludus Romae in agone'), whereas, in all the other narratives, the town gives on to the 'meadow' where bear-hunts and tournaments are held, which attract those who live in the house.

The town and its environs thus constitute the real setting of the narrative. The end of the narrative, which usually comes with the father's departure 'into exile' (N2 and N6), or to the Holy Land (N3, N7 and N9), evokes, but does not describe a distant but indefinite place. This episode does not feature in N1. On the other hand, the knight's castle does not disappear at the end of the narrative as it does in N1.

The action takes place in the distant past: 'jadis' (long ago), 'en antif tans' ('in olden times'), as in N1. The time of year is specified: Whitsuntide (N2 and N6) when 'in accordance with custom' the knight organises a bear-hunt in the 'meadow' or on Trinity Sunday, the first Sunday after Whitsun (N7), the knight going out in the afternoon to a tournament which finishes in the evening. A tournament is also invoked in N3, N4 and N8 to explain the absence of the knight and his family, though in these no precise date is given.

The spatio-temporal setting is different in the two versions of the *Dolopathos* (N10 and N11): the knight and his family have accepted the

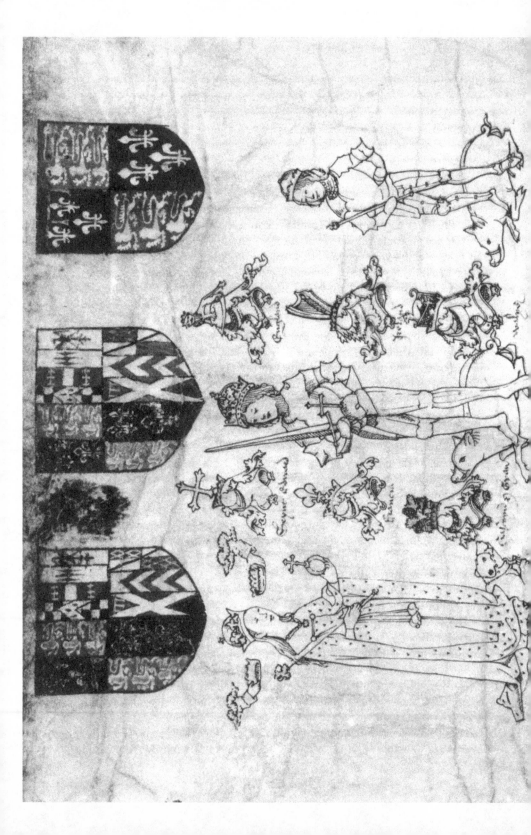

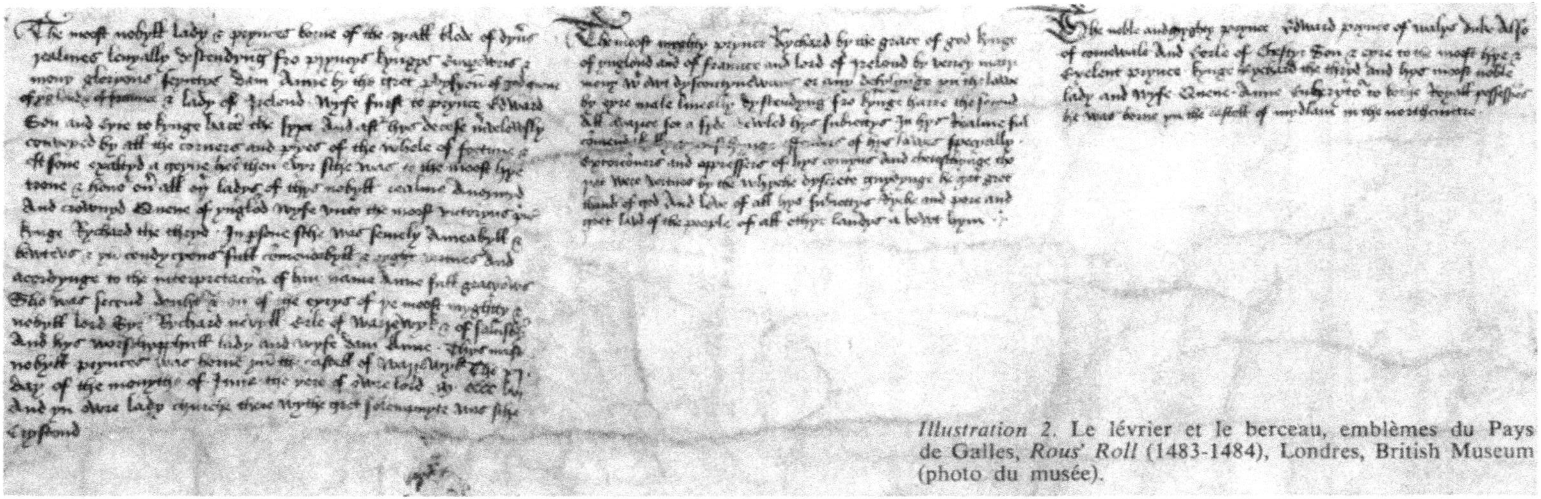

Illustration 2. Le lévrier et le berceau, emblèmes du Pays de Galles, *Rous' Roll* (1483-1484), Londres, British Museum (photo du musée).

2 The greyhound and the cradle, emblems of Wales. *Rous Roll* (1483–4)

hospitality of a citizen near a city, in a large stone house that had remained empty for five years and was situated on the near side of a bridge. It is not the time of year when there are tournaments or ritual bear-hunts, with the bear let loose from its cage for the occasion, but rather the ordinary hunting season. The knight therefore spends every day in the forest in order to feed his family, and it is hunting that accounts for his absence on that particular day. Thus the space of the narrative is not enclosed by the meadow surrounding the town, but gives out on to the game-filled forest. It differs in another respect, too, from the *Roman des sept sages*, in that the knight does not go away at the end, and there is therefore no reference to a place of exile or to a pilgrimage. Nor is the knight's house destroyed, as it is in N1.

Johannes Pauli's version (N12) is in general sparing in its use of detail, but at the end it specifies that the knight enters a Benedictine monastery (which is perhaps equivalent to exile, or the Holy Land, in several of the preceding versions).

2. The actors and the actions
The following characters appear in the reference-narrative:
the father, variously referred to as *dominus* or *miles*;
the child: *puer parvulus*, in the cradle where it sleeps 'soundly' (*suaviter*). One can assume that it is male;
the mother, described from three different perspectives, as the knight's wife (*uxor sua*), as lady (*domina*), and as the child's mother (*mater pueri*);
the nurse;
the snake (*serpens*), which is very big (*maximus*);
the greyhound, often called 'dog'. In the end, its 'usefulness' (*tam utilis*) is recognised;
'divine will'.

The actors combine or are opposed in a number of actions whose sequence in the narrative will be studied later; the chief characteristic of these actions is that, for the most part, each has a corresponding and contrary one, which results in a series of opposite pairs: enter/leave, attack/defend, kill/save, devour/kill, upset/set upright again (i.e., the cradle). Some actions, which are apparently identical, are actually carried out differently: leave at the same time/return one after another; throw (far away)/throw (into the well). Ways of behaving that seem the same result in different actions, which characterise the actors who perform them as mutually opposed. Thus, the women (nurse, then mother) enter, see, believe and *shout out*, whereas the man enters, believes, draws his sword and *kills the greyhound.*

In versions N2 to N9 (*Roman des sept sages* and *Gesta Romanorum*), the actors are as follows:

> the father is a knight, whose valour, nobility, wealth and passion for tournaments are generally emphasised, as is his love for his dog and for his child;
>
> his wife is also 'courtly and wise';
>
> the child, still in the cradle (*infans*), is their only child, born after nine years of barren marriage (N2);
>
> there is not one, but three nurses, whose duties are to bathe him, put him to bed and suckle him, and also, in N8 and N9, to wash his clothes;
>
> the dog is invariably a greyhound, whose age is sometimes specified: five months or thereabouts (N2), one year (N6). His qualities as a hunter are stressed (no prey escapes him), 'quand il prenoit la salvagine yl la tenoit fermement jusques que son maître fut venu' (N4) ('when he caught game he held on to it tightly until his master arrived'), and his talent for anticipating danger: when his master goes to war, the dog holds him back if it has a presentiment of danger threatening him (N3 and N4). The greyhound's faithfulness is always praised and it is called 'the safety and protection of the house' (N8): 'leporarius peroptimus et fidelissimus, salus et protectio hospicii'.
>
> in narratives N3, N4 and N9, the greyhound is accompanied by a falcon (*falco, accipiter*), which is itself a very fine hunter: 'Jamais ne voloit qu'il ne prist quelque proie' ('Never did it fly without catching some prey'). When its master is away it stays on its perch in the child's room.
>
> the snake is described in the greatest detail. In every case it comes out of the old wall in the ruined part of the town, which is its customary haunt. In two cases, N2 and N6, it enters the room through the window.

In all the narratives, the snake is less an enemy from 'outside', as in N1, than an enemy from the borders, from the boundary between outside and inside. It does not come out of the forest, that hunting realm which the knight likes so much. It comes out of the hollows of the wall close by, perhaps from the very depths of the earth. It is described as (N2) 'A wonderfully strong and large snake . . . which had several times, when the earth shook and fissured, been seen to issue forth from its cave . . . Its tail was sharp as a razor, so bad a snake was it' ('Une serpente de merveilleuse force et grandeur . . . qui pluseurs foiz por temps de vainnes ou de mouvemens de terre avoit este veue yssir de sa caverne . . . Sa queue estoit tranchant comme ung raseur, que c'estoit le mauvais serpent'). (The word *vainnes* designates the fissures that open in the earth when it quakes.) N4: 'In a cranny of this castle there was a serpent hidden, of which none knew' ('En ung partuys de cestuy chastiaul avout ung serpent mussé que nul ne sçavoit.') In the title of this text, which would seem to be contemporary with the rest of it, it is called a 'dragon', but the word does not feature in the text itself. N5: 'serpens terribilis et magnus' ('a huge and terrifying snake'); N6: 'un félon serpent sathanas' (a treacherous satanic snake). After it had been cut into pieces by the greyhound, they find 'la teste et l'aguillon, ki molt estoit agus' ('the head and the sting, which was very sharp'). N7: 'le serpens grant et gros, et estoit hideus et porpris de rouse coulor, venimus en toz les manbres de lui' ('the snake was big and fat, quite hideous and coloured red all over, and poisonous in all its limbs'); N8: 'serpens maximus' (a huge snake).

As in the reference-narrative, the unusual size of the snake is emphasised, but it is not a dragon: the one case where that word is used – outside the narrative as such – can only be taken as a sign of the snake's ambiguity. I shall come back to this point below.

The snake is 'treacherous', just as the greyhound is 'faithful'. It is also called Satan. This is not the case in N1, where God ('divine will') is present. N6 is the only narrative in which Satan is explicitly present, N1 the only one in which God is explicitly invoked.

In all the narratives the actions are identical with those in N1, with the exception of a few details and one different ending.

The falcon which features here wakes the greyhound by beating its wings when danger approaches.

The nurses have the same role as in N1, in that they arrive back first, forewarn the mother, who in turn tells the father, but they are specifically said to be *at fault* from the moment they leave the child, which is not the case in N1, and as soon as they see the greyhound they *run away*; in N1, on the other hand, the nurses share in the grief and in the greyhound's funeral.

The knight kills the greyhound, as in N1, but when he returns to the cradle and realises his dreadful mistake, his attitude is noticeably different. Remember that in N1 he grieves with his family and buries the greyhound; the castle is then destroyed by 'divine will' and the estate reduced to a desert. In narratives N2–N9, the knight is just as grief-stricken, but the reasons for his grief are more clearly set out: 'the knight was as woeful as if he had slain a man' ('le chevalier fut tant marry que s'il avoit occis ung homme') (N2). Then he rebukes his wife for having given him bad advice (N3, N4, N5, N7) and even, in N9, has her thrown into prison; he breaks his lance into three (N3, N4, N9), talks of suicide (N4: 'Je me veulx défaire'), commits himself to doing penance (N3: 'A me ipso penitenciam accipiam'; N7: 'Nus ne m'en donra la penance, ge meismes l'en prendrai'), and to that end sets off barefoot and is never seen again (N7: 'Si que nus ne pot savoir où il estoit alez'), or else he goes to spend the rest of his days in the Holy Land (N3, N4, N9). He abandons everything that he holds dear 'sans regarder fame, ne fil, ne heritage, ne or, ne argent' (N7).

For the moment, rather than trying to relate this ending to that of N1, let us consider the differences. The end of the first narrative puts the emphasis on the anxiety of men to preserve the memory of the dead greyhound, and on the intervention of God. The ending of narratives N2–N9 puts the emphasis on the murderer and on the initiative he takes with regard to God by inflicting a penance on himself.

In the two versions of *Dolopathos*, the actors are as follows:

> the father, called a 'youth' (*jeune, juvenis*) or 'squire' in the first part of the narrative (in which he ruins himself and leaves his country), is now called a 'young man' (*bachelier*), or more often a 'knight' (*chevalier, miles*). His only activity is hunting all day with his horse, his greyhound and his falcon, in order to feed his family. He refuses to work with his hands or to beg.
>
> his wife, who has to suckle the baby;
>
> there is no nurse;
>
> the child has just been born;
>
> the greyhound normally goes hunting with his master. Left in the house on this particular day, it is fastened by a chain. Its faithfulness is emphasised;
>
> the falcon and the horse do not themselves do anything;
>
> the snake is very large (*serpens immanis*) and it comes out of the wall of the house, from beneath a large stone, where it lives;
>
> God is not mentioned, either explicitly, as in N1, or implicitly, as in those stories in which the knight imposes a penance upon himself.

The actions represented in the *Dolopathos* differ a little from those in the preceding narratives. The knight does not go to the 'meadow' for a tournament, nor for a bear-hunt. He goes, as ever, to the forest to hunt. The evening before he returned empty-handed, and so on the following day he decides to go out again, but without his dog, which he ties up in the house. He returns loaded down with game.

The mother goes out after he does, because she fears that her child will die of hunger. She goes to a noble lady of the neighbourhood in search of some food. Her departure is not an offence, unlike that of the nurses in N2 and N9, and her quest is not an act of begging, which would have caused her to lose status. The story is quite clear on these two points.

In addition, she returns home *after her husband*, not before him, which means that, unlike the nurses or the mother in the preceding narratives, she has no part in the greyhound's death. Nor does she run away, but goes directly to the cradle, and as soon as she comes in, rights it and without a word suckles and kisses the child (N11):

> L'enfant alète doucement
> Et moult le bèse tendrement.

Where the knight does talk about wanting to die, as in N4, it is when he believes his son to be dead ('Bien voulist estre mis en bière'), and not when he discovers that he has killed his dog unjustly. In his fury he kills not only his dog, but his horse and hawk as well. When his wife discovers the child alive he repents having killed his greyhound, 'but too late'. The same expression was used at the end of the first part of the narrative to describe the feelings of the *juvenis*, as he regretted, 'but too late', that he had squandered his heritage.

There the narrative stops: the knight does not go off on a pilgrimage as in N2–N9, and he does not bury the greyhound, as in N1.

Johannes Pauli's narrative (N12) develops much the same theme, but with much slighter materials. The only characters are:

> the noble (*Edelman, Juncker*);
> his wife;
> the child, still in the cradle;
> the greyhound, which its master loves dearly: 'He would not be parted from it, even for a great sum of money.' As the snake approaches, 'he senses the smell of death';
> the snake, which comes out of the wall.

According to Johannes Pauli, the knight kills his greyhound with his sword ('mit dem Schwert'). But the engraving that accompanies the text in the 1535 edition (illustration 1) shows him hitting the greyhound *with a club*. Neither the text nor the illustration shows the cradle knocked over during the fight. Both documents are in agreement on this point. When he discovers his mistake, the knight leaves, as in N2–N9, but to become a monk. There is no mention of burying the dog. His wife only comes into the narrative at the end, to give him her permission to enter a monastery.

3. The logic of the narrative

The actions that happen during the story are grouped into long narrative sequences in the text (seven in all), which are linked by temporal conjunctions: *cum* (whilst), *autem* (now), *tunc* (then), *ad ultimum* (to conclude).

> 1. 'In diocesi . . . de uxore sua': the spatio-temporal setting
> 2. 'Cum autem exivissent . . . similiter mordentem'

   a. simultaneous exit of the knight, the mother and the nurse
   b. entry of the snake, and assault on the child
   c. greyhound's pursuit of the snake, which knocks over the
      cradle
   d. the snake and the greyhound bite each other
3. 'Quem ad ultimum . . . tractatus'
   a. the greyhound kills the snake
   b. the greyhound throws the snake's body far away
   c. the greyhound waits, covered with blood
4. 'Cum autem intrasset . . . canem occidit'
   a. return of the nurse, who alerts the mother
   b. return of the mother, who alerts the father
   c. return of the father, who kills the dog
5. 'Tunc . . . occisum'
   a. discovery of the child safe and sound
   b. discovery of the snake's body
6. 'Veritatem autem . . . in memoriam facti'
   a. grief of the greyhound's master and mistress
   b. throwing the greyhound's body into the well
   c. burying the body beneath a great pile of stones
   d. planting trees beside the well 'in memory of the dead'
7. 'Castro autem . . . ab habitatore relicto'
   a. destruction of the castle
   b. abandonment of the estate

A simplified plan can be drawn up for the other versions (N2–N9), using italics to indicate the narrative sequences that differ from N1:

   1. spatio-temporal setting
   2. departure of knight and his wife
   3. later and culpable departure of the nurses
   4. entry of snake and assault on the child
   5. *the falcon wakes the greyhound*
   6. pursuit of the snake by the greyhound, which knocks over the
      cradle
   7. death of snake, and concealment of the body
   8. greyhound waits
   9. return of the nurses, who ran away
   10. return of the mother, alerted by the nurses. She alerts the father
   11. return of the father, who kills the dog
   12. righting of the cradle, discovery of the child, safe and sound,
       then of the snake's body
   13. lamentation and *penitential departure of the father*

In the two versions from the *Dolopathos*, the sequence of the narrative is as follows:

1. the knight, *who has returned empty-handed from the hunt the previous evening*, decides to go out without his dog
2. *subsequent departure of the mother, who is afraid her child will die of hunger*
3. entry of snake, and assault on the child
4. pursuit of the snake by the greyhound, which knocks over the cradle
5. greyhound kills the snake
6. *return of the knight first*. He kills the greyhound, *his horse and his falcon*
7. *return of the mother second: she rights the cradle and suckles the child*
8. belated remorse of the father

Finally, in version N12, we have a simpler sequence:

1. introduction to the narrative: a noble had a greyhound that he loved dearly. *The spatial setting is not specified at first*
2. departure of the noble
3. snake comes out of the wall; assault on child
4. the greyhound, sensing the smell of death, attacks and kills the snake
5. when the knight returns, *not having been warned by anything*, he sees the greyhound, but not the snake, hidden beneath the cradle. He kills the greyhound with his sword (text) or *with a club* (engraving)
6. the knight discovers the snake and realises his error
7. lamentations of the knight, *who enters the Benedictine order with the consent of his wife*

The differences between the various narratives now appear in their place in the development of the plot. They concern three moments in the action:

a. The initial departure of the human actors:
either: the knight, the sole human actor, is the only one to go out
or: the nurse goes out at the same time as her master and mistress and without being at fault (N1)
or: the mother goes out after her husband, without being at fault (N10, N11)
or: the nurses go out after the knight and his wife, and are thereby at fault (N2–N9).
b. The return of the human actors:

either: the knight, the sole human actor, comes back alone (N12)

or: the nurse comes back first, alerts the mother, and not being at fault, does not take flight, but shares in the general grief, and attends the dog's funeral (N1)

or: the nurses come back first, alert the mother and, being at fault, take flight (N2–N9)

or: the mother comes back alone, *after the knight* (N10, N11).

c. The end of the narrative:

either: the knight becomes a Benedictine monk (N12)

or: the knight and the other human actors bury the dog in front of the castle, which later disappears (N1)

or: the knight becomes a penitent, leaving his castle and family forever (N2–N9)

or: the knight and his wife are content simply to mourn the dog's death (N10, N11).

If one reads this classification backwards, it emerges that the different possible endings penalise the faults committed or not by the knight, alone or with other actors, either at the moment of departure or at the moment of return. Who, in short, went out culpably, and who legitimately? Who is primarily responsible for the error?

The different permutations are presented in Table 2. If we start at the end, this table enables us first of all to establish a connection between the two types of narrative N2–N9 and N12: in each of them the penitential departure of the knight (whether into exile, or to the Holy Land, or into a monastery) entails the break-up of the family. Then again, the table enables us to oppose type N2–N9 to type N10–N11: in the former, the nurses are responsible for suckling the baby; they are culpable from the moment they leave, which is not the case in any of the other versions; they are the first to return, and they take flight. The narrative finishes with the father's penitential departure and the break-up of the family. In the second, it is the mother who is responsible for feeding the baby; she is not at fault in going out, it is rather that she is concerned to find food so that she can suckle her child; she returns *after* her husband, and therefore had nothing to do with the greyhound's death, and far from taking flight, she immediately suckles her son. The narrative concludes on a new note of stability, and not with the father's departure and the separation of the members of the family. This comparison establishes a connection between a fault that may be committed by the woman responsible for suckling the child, and the ending of the narrative. What is the connection in the reference-narrative?

The nurse is responsible for the child. Like the mother in N10–N11, the nurse in N1 does not commit a fault by going out, but unlike her, she comes back before the others and leads them into error, as in N2–N9. This

			N 10–11	N 1	N 2–9	N 12
Departure	wrongful (of the nurses)				▓	
	not wrongful	of the nurses		▓		
		of the mother (in the absence of the nurses)	▓			
		of the knight (the only person present)				▓
The one most responsible for the mistake	the knight	in the absence of his wife				▓
		his wife having come back after him	▓			
	the nurse or nurses		▓	▓	▓	
End of the narrative	penitential departure of the knight: consequent destruction of the family				▓	▓
	funeral of the greyhound, destruction of the castle, and abandonment of the estate			▓	▓	
	simple regret		▓			

Table 2 *The logic of the narrative*

narrative is thus both close to N2–N9 and N10–N11, and different from them, as is confirmed by the ending, which is unlike the others, though closer to the first type than the second: there is no new stability, but eventual destruction for the *castrum*. The burial of the dog can be linked with the penitential behaviour in N2–N9 and N12, so long as an essential difference is emphasised: the *peasant* story in the *exemplum* places the emphasis on remembering the victim, not on the murderer's repentance, and on the transcendent intervention of 'divine will' rather than on the knight's initiative.

Content analysis

As before, I shall survey in turn the spatio-temporal setting, the principal actors and the actions that link them, but this time I shall consider them in terms of the meaning that they must have had in the culture of their time.

All the versions, including the peasant legend from the *exemplum*, place the action in contemporary chivalric society. The action almost invariably unfolds in a castle, albeit fictionalised, which is lived in by the knight, his lady, his nurses, and the heir to the lineage. Their occupations are those of the lay aristocracy: 'games' like bear-hunting and, particularly, tournaments, which were in fact usually held at Whitsuntide, after the young knights had been dubbed.[27] The other aristocratic activities were hunting and war, both of which are mentioned in the narratives.

What place did the greyhound, the hero of all these narratives, occupy in this society?

One should first of all bear in mind that, generally speaking, dogs were somewhat disparaged in the Middle Ages, while greyhounds on the other hand were highly valued. Vincent of Beauvais, in the mid thirteenth century, distinguished three sorts of dogs: hunting dogs, with long drooping ears, guard dogs, which are 'more rustic than other dogs', and greyhounds, which by contrast are 'the noblest, the most elegant, the swiftest, and the best at hunting'.[28]

In chivalric society, the greyhound was also an emblem, often found on tombs, at the feet of the effigies of gentlemen, where it symbolised the chivalric virtues (faith), occupations (hunting) and, more generally, the whole aristocratic way of life. It is quite clear that, where tombs are concerned, the greyhound is always associated with knighthood – along with the lion, symbolising strength – and never with ladies, who are generally associated with the little lap-dog, symbol of conjugal fidelity and domestic virtue.[29]

This throws some light on the knight's crime, and emphasises its seriousness: the knight kills the animal that incarnates his own system of values, and is a kind of double of himself or of the son who is destined one day to succeed him. Thus the greyhound's *fides*, its faith in the feudal sense of the term, is emphasised in almost all the stories.

The greyhound finds its opposite in the snake. The word (*serpent*) is ambiguous, as it can be used to mean both a whole family of reptiles and one of those reptiles in particular. Isidore of Seville's chapter 'De serpentibus' includes the marine *anguis*, the snake (*serpens*) that lives on land, the 'lustful' grass-snake (*coluber*) and the dragon which flies through the air.[30] In the thirteenth century, Gervaise's *Bestiaire* distinguishes three sorts of serpents, viper, grass-snake, dragon.[31]

Our stories depict a snake in the strict sense, and not a dragon, as is confirmed by his living on land, and not in the air, and by the fact that he bites the greyhound: according to Isidore, the strength of snakes lies in their teeth, of dragons in their tails. There is some uncertainty, admittedly, in the stories; the title of one of them has 'dragon' instead of 'snake', but it is a snake nonetheless, and not a dragon of the sort that so many saints have to face in hagiographic accounts. The snake in the *exemplum* resembles neither Tarasque, who was subdued by Saint Martha, nor the dragon vanquished by Saint Marcellus of Paris.[32]

One of the texts most often quoted in connection with snakes in the Middle Ages was Genesis 3, 1: 'The serpent was more subtle than any beast of the field' (Raban Maur, Hugh of Saint-Victor, Petrus Comestor, Vincent of Beauvais). It is cold and humid by nature.[33] These two qualities explain how it lives on land, which is cold and dry, distinct from water (cold and wet like the serpent), air (hot and wet) and fire (hot and dry).[34]

Because of its nature, the snake is vulnerable to cold. This is why it buries itself in rocks or hollow trees during winter. Similarly, it is less harmful at night, because of the cold. It prefers to come out in the daytime, and in the spring: 'Verno tempore prodeunt', says Vincent of Beauvais in the thirteenth century.

Our texts bear this out, for the snake comes out at Whitsun, in the afternoon (N7).

Again, in nineteenth-century folklore, people were fearful of the snake's emergence at the beginning of the May rituals: in some regions, a small tree or leafy branch was planted in a dunghill to prevent the snakes from coming to suck the cows' udders.[35]

In most of our stories, the snake comes out of a hollow in an old wall. According to Hildegard of Bingen, the snake tries to find shade among the stones in order to protect it from the sun's heat.[36] A whole tradition, discernible in bestiaries as well as in our stories, shows snakes living in the hollows of old walls.[37]

One of our narratives specifies the snake's colour. It is red, or, more specifically, crimson. This is a well-known colour in medieval literature, and was also used in vestments, in the symbolism of kingship, and in heraldry.[38] Philip of Thaün argues that purple symbolises Christ's passion.[39] But it is the colour's origin that is significant here. According to Vincent of Beauvais, a ray of sunlight (hot) passing through water vapour (humid) gives the clouds a 'flame-red [colour] which is known as crimson'.[40] And our snake, who has the same characteristics as water, surely derives his colour from the hot and humid vapours which shake the earth's interior.

Indeed, in another story, it is said that the snake customarily comes out of its retreat when there are earth-tremors. These earth-tremors would be produced by disturbance of the water vapours in the bowels of the earth. For the vapours to escape it must be both very humid and very hot, which is why earth-tremors are rare in summer and winter, when the weather is either too dry or too cold, and why, on the other hand, they are common in the rainy season of autumn, or – as in our text – in spring.[41]

The Christian symbolism of the snake is not given much weight in the stories, the only explicit reference being in N6, where the serpent is compared to the *félon serpent Sathanas* (wicked serpent Satan). This reference can be placed within the Genesis tradition, or more accurately, within that of the Book of Revelation, when the dragon, also called 'that old serpent', prepares to devour a newly born child; while the mother flees into the wilderness, Saint Michael intervenes with the help of his angels and the dragon is thrown to the earth (Revelation, 12, 1–9). Like the serpent in one of our stories, the dragon–serpent of Revelation is called 'the Devil, and Satan' (12, 9). Medieval representations preserve this same ambiguity, with the emphasis sometimes falling on the dragon aspect, sometimes on the serpent. But in neither case is there any doubt about its diabolic nature: the full meaning of the danger threatening the child, and the momentous nature of the combat between greyhound and serpent, have thus become apparent.

The knight also has a crucial part to play in these narratives. By his very title, and by his activities (hunting, war, tournaments), he represents the chivalric ethic; it is out of fear of being dishonoured that the *juvenis* leaves the country and sets out to make a new life elsewhere, while still eschewing work or begging as 'rustic' occupations unworthy of the noble hunter (N10–N11). Now, the knight kills the greyhound which is 'faithful' to him, in contrast to the serpent which is 'treacherous'. By committing a murderous 'injustice' against the faithful greyhound, which causes him to weep 'as if it had been a man', the knight becomes as 'wicked' as the serpent. This is how one should interpret the sixteenth century engraving: the Junker is holding a club, not a sword, in other words the weapon of wild, uncivilised man. Allowances have of course to be made for the aesthetic fashions of German Renaissance art, in which wild men abound. But this detail also makes it clear that the knight's murderous gesture implies a negation of his own ethic, which is tantamount to a rejection of culture and a return to the wild state. Only the penitential departure (in this case to a monastery, in others to the

Holy Land) can redeem his guilt, although it cannot restore him to his native milieu, since he 'is dead to the world'. In version N12, and in the engraving accompanying it, the character of the knight thus passes through three different states in the course of the narrative:

Knight	Murderer	Monk
=	=	=
master of the castle	wild man	dead to the world

In this version we are not told the time of year at which the murder takes place, but it is worth noting that folk tradition, especially in Germany, depicts the 'emergence' of the wild man in spring, or more precisely, at Shrovetide Carnival or Whitsun.[42] The action in several of the versions in the *Roman des sept sages* also takes place then.

Our analysis of the narrative's logic has shown the question of suckling the child, and of the role of the nurses (in versions N1–N9), to be fundamental to it. More specifically, the absence or presence or the degree of seriousness that attaches to the nurses' fault dictate the choice of different 'possible narratives'. The 'morality' of nurses was in fact a major preoccupation in the domestic ethics of the aristocracy of this period. A passage in the *Roman des sept sages* deplores the fact that nurses are no longer chosen as carefully as they used to be, and the danger that the baleful influence of unworthy milk 'may debase the lineage':

> Lors estoit droite la lignie
> Mais or est forment abaissie
> . . .
> Quant un haus home a un enfant
> Son fils courtois et avenant
> Lors devroit une gentil femme
> Querre entour lui partout le regne
> Se li fesist l'enfant bailler
> Pour bien norrir et ensaigner . . .[43]

> (Then was the lineage noble, but now it is much debased... When a noble man has a child, his son courtly and comely, then should a 'gentil' woman be sought throughout the kingdom to look after him [if the child is going to be wet-nursed], to ensure that he is nourished and brought up properly.)

The end of the reference-story deserves special attention. The burial of the unjustly killed greyhound comprises several stages. First, its body is thrown into the well *in front of* the castle door. This door plays an important part in the narratives, for through it the human actors leave or enter the castle. In N2 the nurses take the precaution of 'shutting the door (*l'uys*) of the room'. In N10 the knight has received lodging from the citizen, in a

house that has been untenanted for five years, and is given the door key by
the host himself. Conversely, the serpent seems never to enter by the door: it
comes out of a hole in the castle wall, or else enters *by the window* if it has
first gone out through a gap in the town wall. The serpent avoids or
circumvents the door, but never passes through it. In all Indo-European
societies, the door embodies the division between outside and inside and, as
Benveniste points out, the same word, *foris*, was used to mean both 'door'
and 'outside'.[44] In our narratives, the castle door effects a material division
between domestic and external space, and shields the former from the
dangers of the latter. This is why the serpent cannot use the door. In N7, the
town gate, with its drawbridge, also separates urban space from the 'sub-
urban' space of chivalric games. There are as many doors as there are areas
concentrically arranged around the *domus*. In the reference-narrative, there
is no further horizon to set off the violent opposition between the inside and
the outside of the house. Now, the greyhound is buried near the door, but
outside the house: the 'memory' of its death is thus dissociated from the
castrum, which is doomed to disappear, and thereby enabled to endure.

The greyhound's body was thrown into the well and covered with a great
pile of stones. Trees were then planted beside the well. It is not easy to
provide a complete interpretation of this complex motif. Throwing the body
into the well, then stoning it, may suggest that the knight, already
responsible for the greyhound's death, is doing the victim's body a new
injustice by treating it so ignominiously. This hypothesis is the more
plausible if one recalls that wells often stood for the mouth of hell, as for
instance in the apocryphal legend of Pontius Pilate, who committed suicide,
and whose body was thrown, first into the Tiber, then into the Rhône, where
its mere presence was enough to cause storms and floods. To be rid of this
evil corpse, they threw it into an Alpine lake or, according to an illumination
in a Milanese manuscript, into a well. This represents the mouth of hell, for
self-murder is punished by eternal damnation.[45] Moreover, throwing down
a well and stoning were ignominious punishments in the thirteenth century:
on 3 May 1211, after Simon de Montfort and the army of the Albigensian
crusade had taken the castle of Lavaur, Giraude of Lavaur, the lady of the
castle and a reputedly dangerous heretic, was thrown down a well, which
was then filled with stones. William of Tudèle, who was less opposed to the
Albigensians than other chroniclers, deplored this punishment, which in his
eyes was 'a tragedy and a crime'.[46]

. But this episode is not identical to the motif that concerns us, for Giraude
of Lavaur was thrown into the well while still alive, whereas in our narrative
it is a corpse that is thrown in. In both cases, filling it up with stones is linked
to the total destruction (military in one case, supernatural in the other) of a
castle tainted by crime (heresy in one case, unjust murder in the other), and
to the prevention of any permanent occupation of the land through blocking

of the water-source. But it is only in the second case that trees are planted beside the well, and how is one to account for the tears of the knight and his family if the fate of the greyhound's body is as negative as the punishment inflicted on the lady of Lavaur? Rather than compounding his offence, the knight seems to repent of the injustice he has done and to carry out a positive funeral rite. Do other narratives or practices confirm this hypothesis?

Wells can have more than one meaning; they do not always, for instance, represent the mouth of hell. Our legend should be compared with those told of various holy martyrs whose bodies, or parts of them, were thrown into wells, as, for example, Saint Valerian in the crypt of the church of Saint Philibert of Tournus, or Saint Bausange at Saint-Pierre-et-Saint-Bausange (Aube).[47] If this comparison is justified, the greyhound's burial, followed by the planting of the trees, predicts the peasants' worship of the greyhound, in the legend itself. There is a fundamental difference, however, for with Saint Valerian and Saint Bausange the wells remain in use and the presence of the holy bodies gives their water healing properties. In Saint Guinefort's case, the description of the rite no longer mentions the well, as if the accumulation of stones thrown on to the body had been big enough (*maximus*) to fill the well in completely. But this is never explicitly stated, and trees are planted beside (*juxta*) the well, as if it were still open. But it is surely preferable to adopt the hypothesis that the well was filled in, for this would foreshadow the abandonment of the estate that is mentioned shortly afterwards in the legend. In addition, the great pile of stones that covers the greyhound's body suggests a specific folk ritual, the building of *mergers* or *murgers*. These were heaps of stones reputed to have been built up gradually in order to preserve the memory of a dead man, and local legends generally present them as tombs.[48]

Planting trees 'in memory of the dead' can also be linked with a motif from oral tradition, namely 'the magic tree on the tomb' studied by Vladimir Propp. In his essay, Propp derives this motif from the propitiatory rites of hunting cultures (often some of the game killed was buried under a tree to ensure plentiful supply in the future) and farming cultures (where a similar ritual ensured that the fruit trees would bear a good crop). Evidence from the sixteenth century in France shows that burying a dead dog under a dying tree was still believed to give the tree strength and to rejuvenate it.[49] In each case, the tree growing above the corpse would symbolise life springing up after death. This is why the motif was easily assimilated to Christianity: it is not uncommon to find a tree growing above a martyr's tomb in the hagiographic legends of the late Middle Ages.[50]

The narrative of the greyhound's burial, in its complex form, is thus related to rites, beliefs and oral folk traditions concerned with the worship of the dead, and more particularly with the worship of the holy martyrs.

After the burial of the greyhound, 'the castle was destroyed by divine will and the estate, reduced to a desert, was abandoned by its inhabitants'.

This can be read in two different ways. Either the ruin and depopulation happened through the will of God, though without being in any way a divine punishment; in which case the peasants were simply stating facts, and invoking the will of God as explanation. Or else God wanted thereby to punish the knight for his crime.

The second hypothesis seems preferable, for the majority, if not all, of the many medieval traditions concerning destruction and depopulation are in fact associated with supernatural punishments, curses, anathema or excommunication. A number of Stephen of Bourbon's *exempla* confirm this point. Thus, a chivalric lineage is obliterated after an excommunication, and a castle is abandoned. Elsewhere, cities cursed long ago by Charlemagne have since then been 'reduced to wilderness and abandoned by all their inhabitants'. Likewise, a priest excommunicates an orchard where young people were wont to pick apples on a Sunday, and the orchard becomes barren. Stephen of Bourbon is surprised by the barrenness of a forest near Belley and by the dearth of fish in a pond, whereupon the local people explain that a local priest has placed both forest and pond under an anathema, because a knight had taken them from the monks.[51] The consequences are identical in the greyhound narrative, but they proceed directly from 'divine will'; no form of curse, or, more significantly, excommunication from the church, is uttered. This helps to explain why ecclesiastical excommunication should have been so effective, for it struck a chord in folk culture which made it all the more credible, so much so in fact that lay people sometimes reinforced the clerics' confidence in their own formulae.[52]

There is another reason for interpreting the destruction of the castle and the depopulation of the estate as a divine punishment. Killing one's dog, in folk culture, is an act fraught with consequences. In Provence it brings seven years' bad luck.[53] And a seventeenth-century proverb has it that 'killing his dog brings misfortune either to the murderer or to someone living in his house'.[54]

Now, in this version God's punishment appears all the more severe for allowing no appeal. In versions N2–N9, the knight takes the initiative by his penitence, and can hope to gain a pardon from God through his pilgrimage. In our version, on the other hand, it is God's will that is operative, rather than that of the knight. And even if the murderer is careful to bury his victim in such a way as to perpetuate his memory, the lord's castle and estate do not escape the divine anger.

The originality of the peasant version

It was not my intention, in conducting a comparative analysis of the different versions of the narrative, to confuse them but rather to highlight their differences. I have thus come to the conclusion that the reference narrative differs significantly from the others, and at a number of crucial points.

N1 is the only version that stems from the peasant oral tradition. All the others are taken from written works belonging to learned culture. However, it is important to remember that even in this case all we have is a written text, part of learned culture, an *exemplum*, with its own special rules of composition. It is therefore hard to decide which parts of the narrative belong to the oral tradition, and which may be attributed to a genre peculiar to learned culture.

The *exemplum* says 'the same thing' as the other narratives, particularly N2–N9, but tends to do it in a remarkably economical way. There is one nurse, rather than two or three; there is just a greyhound, and no falcon; the snake 'enters', but we are not told where it 'comes out of'; it is described as 'very big', but no further details are given; the cradle is knocked over during the struggle, but the narrator omits to say that it is righted again, although this would have to be the case if the child were ever to be discovered.

If there is only one nurse, and if there is no falcon, this may well mean that the *exemplum* represents the chivalric milieu from the point of view of someone living in a peasant cottage. This model would comprise a lord, his lady, their son (who would be the sole heir), a nurse and a greyhound. But it is in the nature of an *exemplum* to be schematic, and it may therefore have reduced the number of characters.

Space is treated in a particularly remarkable manner in this narrative. I would, in fact, argue that the literary genre of *exemplum* does not usually require such detail, and that here it must really be the voice of the peasants that we hear.

The other versions generally begin by locating the action fairly vaguely 'at Rome', 'in a city', etc. This *exemplum* is much more precise, in that it specifies the diocese, the nearest village, and the current lord of the estate where the events took place. This detail may be said to be a characteristic feature of *exempla*, for they were meant to be presented in as authentic a form as possible: what 'trustworthy' informant has told the author of the *exemplum* the narrative he is recounting? Where and when did the author encounter the events from which he has drawn the *exemplum*? But this is not a complete explanation, for the peasant legend too has to root itself as exactly as possible in geographical space, in that it is tied to a particular cult site.

The end of the narrative confirms this. In all the other versions, we find no physical trace of the events that have occurred. The knight himself often disappears, nobody ever sees him again, and no one knows the country of his destination. N1, however, ends with the earth itself preserving on its actual surface a memory of the events, and where the greyhound was once so unjustly killed, there is now a wood that conceals a tomb in the middle of a 'desert'.

It is easy enough to account for this variant ending. All the other narratives derive from improving works whose function is to persuade the reader or the listener to forbear from acting rashly and, in some cases, from listening to his wife's advice, or from succumbing to blind anger. Johannes Pauli concludes his narrative as follows:

> In the town where these events took place it is now forbidden to embark upon anything important without first having reflected upon it three times and discussed it in Council. So that nothing should be done in too much haste, others have ordered that people should recite the twenty-four letters of the alphabet before acting, as the Emperor Theodosius should have done when he was banished by Saint Ambrose for rashly causing so much blood to be spilled.

But the peasant legend recorded by Stephen of Bourbon has no such 'moral' appended to it. From the start it is located in a defined place, and its actual unfolding involves a reordering of appearances, such that it claims to lay the material basis for a rite which is a logical extension of it.

The ending of the peasant legend bears the unmistakable imprint of folk culture. The semantic analysis of other parts of the narrative required us to draw on a wide range of information from clerical and learned culture (the Bible, encyclopaedias, bestiaries) or from aristocratic lay culture (hunting manuals), but this last episode, by contrast, can only be understood in the context of peasant culture, and indeed with respect to our more recent knowledge of it.

At the start of this analysis, I raised the question of the 'origin' of the peasant legend: was it autochthonous, or should one invoke the dual-diffusion hypothesis (diffusion of an oriental narrative, the popularisation of a learned narrative)? Which of these alternatives ought one to adopt? The general characteristics of N1 most resemble those of N2–N9, and it would therefore be justifiable to argue that a popularisation of the learned narrative occurred in the second half of the twelfth century, even if we cannot know all the attendant circumstances. But the influence of folk, or more particularly peasant, culture is nevertheless very marked. It has served to root the legend in local geography, to enrich it with a variety of folklore motifs, and to link it inseparably with a healing rite. There would therefore be no point in setting the two hypotheses up as alternatives, for, far from being irreconcilable, each clearly tells a part of the truth.

5

THE RITE

At the beginning of the *exemplum*, Stephen of Bourbon cites two instances of the kind of idolatry he is condemning. He writes of superstitious women casting lots in order to treat children, some of whom 'adore' elder plants and make offerings to them, whilst others take sick children to anthills or 'other things'. The inquisitor regards both of these practices as being identical in kind with those he suppressed at the cult site of Saint Guinefort.

There is plenty of evidence in more recent folklore for the healing powers of elder. It is used to cure cattle, or to keep snakes that suck milk away from cows. Elder flowers are also good for human beings. 'The elder is a doctor', they used to say in Upper Brittany, and each flower was held to be the refuge of a fairy. The plant is also associated with witchcraft; it wards off spells, and beating witches with elder rods hurts them more than other kinds of wood; it also has evil powers of its own, so that touching an animal with an elder stick may cause it to die, and using the wood to make fires may stop hens laying. It is also insulting to point a flowering branch of elder at a girl, as it is an accusation of duplicity or fickle behaviour.[1]

Anthills have the same sort of powers. It is important to avoid kicking them over or destroying them, else you risk having your cattle die shortly afterwards. Although insects play a much less important part in folk medicine than plants, anthills are often used to cure beasts or men. An egg is placed on top of one, and when the ants have finished eating it, the sick person is cured. To win the favours of the woman you love, you have to put a frog in a box full of holes and put it in the anthill: when the frog is completely devoured, the spell will have done its work.[2]

The rite performed on the supposed tomb of Saint Guinefort resembles these practices. But the *exemplum* makes it clear that they are not to be confused. There would be no justification, for instance, for arguing that the small trees which are next mentioned in the text are elders.

The description that Stephen of Bourbon gives, which is derived from information he himself received, allows us to analyse the nature of the ritual space, the final purpose of the pilgrimage, and the sequence of the rite. The cult site (*locus*) is 'a league' away from a *castrum*. At this period, that can only mean a 'French league' (also known as a *lieue de terre* and a *lieue commune*, a league of land and a common league), which is found in documents from the twelfth century onwards, and which was the equivalent of 4.440 kilometres.[3] It is in the diocese of Lyons, 'near' Neuville-les-Dames, called *villa* (village?), and it is on the banks of the Chalaronne, a small tributary of the Saône, about six kilometres from Neuville-les-Dames as the crow flies. The fact that this distance is substantially more than a French league, and the use of the term *villa* for Neuville-les-Dames, means that this cannot be the site of the *castrum* where the mothers went to find the witch.

The term *castrum* is imprecise. Here it probably refers to a village or to a small fortified town with a mixed population, in which a witch is said to live. In the legend I have translated it as 'castle' (*château*), for the only people mentioned as living there belong to the lord's family. But it could also mean 'fortified town'.

The place of pilgrimage is wooded, but the types of small tree and bush are not specified. This wood is said to have grown up on the site of a *castrum*, near to its well, both of which have now disappeared. It is separate from the forest (*silva*), out of which wolves come, and in which fauns dwell. The name of the forest, *Rimite*, can no longer be traced in local place names.[4] We cannot therefore at present locate the wood more precisely, but the name is itself an interesting one. It belongs to the same family as the word *heremitas*, which in the Middle Ages designates uncultivated land, the refuge of hermits (*eremita*). This forest is, as its name suggests, a 'desert' in the medieval sense of the term. It is a forest, and the abode of wild beasts (wolves) and ambiguous powers which affect the beings that live there ('fauns' and wild men on the one hand, holy hermits on the other). Between the tenth and thirteenth centuries the forest was tackled by settlers, but with varied success and for various lengths of time, for clearances and desertions go hand in hand. The name of the forest, *Rimite*, should therefore be considered in connection with the place name *Noville* (Neuville-les-Dames), which implies a recent settlement, and in connection with the peasants' oral tradition, with its reference to the desertion of a *castrum*.

The cult site, comprising a wood and a river, is placed halfway between a fortified town, permanently inhabited by man, and the forest, the abode of wolves and fauns. People living on either side visit it from time to time; the witch, and the mothers who went to seek her out, come from the *castrum* to perform rites, while the wolves, on the other hand, are liable to emerge from the forest and carry off children, and the mothers adjure the fauns to leave their wild haunts for a moment to come to this place. It thus appears to be an intermediate space in which from time to time nature and culture come into contact with each other. There are two categories of pilgrim who visit this cult site. There are those generally described as 'peasants' (*homines rusticani*) who come because of 'their infirmities and their needs'. Their specific purposes are left as vague as their identities, and they only make up a small proportion of the pilgrim body. The pilgrimage is efficacious for a variety of ailments, but it is especially and primarily concerned with children.

Stephen of Bourbon's *exemplum* is entirely concerned with children. Thus, the first narrative tells of a *puer* still in the cradle, while the account of the rite likewise describes *pueri*, who must be equally young, since they are carried by their mothers. Does the term *puer* designate a specific age? It is not customarily used to mean infants or very young children, yet there cannot be any doubt that they are the *pueri* here described. The classic vocabulary of the *Ages of Life*, transmitted by Isidore of Seville and Gregory the Great, generally distinguishes between *infantia* (up to seven years old), *pueritia* (from seven to fourteen years old) and *adolescentia* (from fourteen to twenty-one years old),[5] This, albeit with some variations, was the dominant usage in the Middle Ages, and Stephen of Bourbon himself uses it when he describes himself as a *puer*, when he was a schoolboy in the schools of Saint Vincent of Mâcon.[6] At Montaillou, in the early fourteenth century, in a peasant community comparable with the one described in the text of the *exemplum*, a young child was not yet called *puer* (which designates a child between the ages of two and twelve years), but *infans* (unable to speak), and yet more often, *filius* or *filia* (depending on the sex).[7] The two words *infans* and *filius* are used in similar fashion in some of the narratives parallel to the legend. In the latter, however, the sex of the child is not specified. In the first narrative, the word clearly has to be taken in the restricted sense of 'male baby', the heir to a chivalric line. This may well be the case with the rite also, but we cannot be certain.

It is equally hard to know for certain from which diseases the children suffered. They are described as being 'feeble and sick', or 'sick and weak', and thin too, since their mothers hope to find them 'fat and well' when they reclaim them. There is no reason to be surprised by this vagueness regarding the children's health, for, even with adults joining pilgrimages that were most closely supervised by the church, medieval descriptions seldom lend themselves to a modern clinical interpretation. Imprecision is all the more common in the case of children, which serves to show yet again how undeveloped the 'idea of childhood' was in the Middle Ages.[8] Children's illnesses are hardly described in even the most informed of medieval medical books. The first fleeting references we have to the illnesses suffered by ill-nourished and neglected children are to be found in a work of a very different order, the late thirteenth-century manual of education by Ramon Lull: they suffer from ringworm, their hair falls out and they are covered in abscesses ('enfants tigneus et pleins de apostumes'), they catch the plague and scrofula ('les enfants en deviennent esglandeuls et escroelés et (ont) moult d'autres maladies').[9] However, more recent evidence from folklore suggests that other maladies are more likely, children's complaints which are nowadays thought to be mild but which would then probably have had rapid and severe consequences, such as rickets or simply slowness in learning to walk.

The rite may be broken down into three separate sequences, each of which was scrupulously controlled by the witch.

It begins with some preliminaries, namely the offering of salt and other unspecified things (bread? coins?). I have no intention of treating this gift as an example of the 'universal symbolism' of salt which Ernest Jones thought he had discovered, and for which he provided a psychoanalytic interpretation.[10] The gift of salt needs to be considered in the specific symbolic context that this ritual provides. Some of Jones's conclusions are nonetheless pertinent here: the ambivalence of salt, which can equally well attract demons and witches as cause them to take flight, the frequent association of water and fire with salt, as in the baptismal rite, or in the casting of spells (for example, throwing salt on the fire).

Once these offerings had been made, the children's swaddling-clothes were hung on bushes and nails were driven into the trunks of the trees that were supposed to have grown above the dog's tomb. A relationship is thus established between the sick body and the body of the 'martyr', through the intermediate agencies of the clothes, the nails, the wood and the roots of the trees.

The crucial feature of the rite's central sequence is the temporary separation of the mother and child, and the supposed intervention of the fauns.

To begin with, the mother and the witch stand on either side of the two trees and pass the child nine times backwards and forwards between them. While they are doing this, they also speak, requesting the fauns to take back this child, who i sick and belongs to them, and to return their own child, in good health, whom they had stolen. We thus learn that a first substitution had taken place without the women's knowledge. The function of the rite is to bring about a second, reverse, substitution to restore things to their proper state, with the women recovering their children, and the fauns likewise. The intermediate position of the cult site, between nature and culture, is clearly appropriate to a rite whose basic function is one of exchange.

But the performance of the rite requires specific conditions, which are prescribed in the most meticulous detail: the child placed at the foot of the tree is naked, as at birth; he is going back to his parents, the fauns, just as his double, returned by the fauns, is, in his mother's eyes, being reborn.

The mothers have to be separated from their children for the substitution to take place. The distance and duration of this separation are carefully measured: the distance is as far as the infants' cries will carry (they must be out of earshot and out of sight), and the duration is that in which a candle takes to burn out. The candle very probably serves as something more than an instrument for measuring time, for, being fire, it must play a crucial part, in relation to the salt offered in the first phase of the cult and to the local vegetation, in the symbolic system of the cult.

The presence of fire also allows the women to emphasise the risk the child runs in being left alone. The narrative tells of children being burned and sometimes dying, but even though this is described as an accident, the witnesses themselves say that it happened a number of times, and I would therefore argue that it was an integral part of the rite.[11] This is also the case with the threat of the wolf, which sometimes emerges from the forest instead of the fauns, and devours the child. But the wolf is the devil, just as the faun is a demon. The clerical exegesis affirms this, but on the basis of the women's evidence: the abandonment of the child leaves the mother alone and at the mercy of terrifying demonic forces. Inasmuch as the fire and the wolf threaten to devour the child, the rite may be said to be a test.

If, therefore, the women address invocations to the fauns, it is because the rite involves the dangerous conjunction of two hostile worlds. Will the fauns, who have stolen their children, agree to return them? Will the child survive the test? In order for the exchange to take place, humans and demons, women and fauns, culture and wild nature must for a moment come together over the child, who will not in every case be able to escape from them. And even if the child is still alive when the mother returns to it, which child is it, the child of men or of fauns?

The rite's final sequence provides an answer to this question. After the test comes the proof. If the child dies, the fauns have not consented to take back their sick child. If he survives, however, that is proof that he is the healthy human child restored by the fauns. The rite thus comes to a close, with a symmetrical resolution in which the nine immersions into the running water of the river correspond to the nine times the child was passed between the trees. It also completes the symbolic pattern by which the hot and the dry of the earlier part of the rite, under the sign of the fire, is opposed by, and is superseded by, the cold and wet of the river water.

Before proceeding any further with the interpretation of the ritual, I shall identify all the sequences of the rite that have been analysed. Each element, considered in isolation, is familiar to folklorists. Thus, one comparable and widely attested practice involves the placing of a sick child's body, or just his head, in a cavity which gives on to a place known for its therapeutic powers. There is also the custom of passing a child a particular number of times between the forks of a cleft tree, or between two small trees that, half way up, have grown together.[12]

The draping of children's clothes over bushes, and the driving of nails into the bark of trees, are also well known. In both cases, the idea is to rid the body of its illness and to transfer it, by contact, to plants.[13] It is not a 'tree cult', such as were denounced by Councils in the early Middle Ages. In recent folk practice, and in the *exemplum* too, trees are merely instrumental to the rite; pilgrims praying to the saint of a chapel may also hang their sick children's clothes on a nearby tree, but that does not mean that they are venerating the tree. The same goes for the women, who make their appeal to demons and fauns, not to trees.

Yet, at the time that the garments are placed on the bushes, the cure has not yet happened, it is still only anticipated. The clothes, swaddling-clothes, shoes or whatever have often been interpreted as *ex votos*, but as they are gathered up again after the rite at the pilgrimage site, they are strictly speaking preliminaries to the cure, not tokens of gratitude.[14]

There is a wealth of recent, even current, evidence for these practices. Is the same true of the Middle Ages, particularly in the Dombes? In 1158 the Cluniac monks of the Priory of Gigny, in the Jura, processed through the Dombes carrying the reliquary of Saint Taurinus, in an attempt to collect sufficient funds to rebuild their church, for it had been destroyed by fire. Among other places, they stopped at Neuville-les-Dames, which is mentioned a century later in our text. Reading between the lines, this document can be said to reveal several local folk practices: at Bâgé, the shrine was placed at the foot of an old oak tree that stood in the centre of a field, and a paralytic was straightway cured. He gave thanks to Saint Taurinus while the people divided the branches of the oak among themselves and bore them off in the hope that they would help them in the future.[15] The monastic worship of the saint is here mingled with the folk worship of an oak tree. It is a surprisingly ambiguous situation, clearly fostered by the monks of Gigny in order to extend the worship of Saint Taurinus.

The famous treatise that Archbishop Agobard of Lyons (who lived from 779 to 840) wrote against superstition is yet earlier, but he unfortunately only denounces one particular type of belief and practice: that of the *tempestarii*, who foretold storms and could ward off hail and thunder. Agobard says nothing about healing rites.[16]

But if we are concerned to define normative texts for this period, we can go beyond the strictly regional framework. Bishop Burchard of Worms, at the beginning of the eleventh century, imposed a year of penitence on mothers who put their children 'on the roof or in a hole' in the hope of ridding them of fever, and – like many others – denounces the worship of trees, stones and fountains, forbidding candles to be burned at them or offerings to be made.[17]

It is enough to note how ancient and how enduring these practices were. It would be pointless, however, to speculate as to their 'pagan origins', as the medieval clergy did and as nineteenth-century folklorists have done. They did undoubtedly date from before the spread of Christianity, but we apprehend them only in a Christian context, and the *exemplum* clearly shows how far they are integrated with the beliefs and rites of Christians in the thirteenth century. Their place in the religion of these peasants is a genuine problem, but the question of their 'origins' can only give rise to idle speculations.

The rite's central sequence illustrates another belief that is familiar to folklorists, namely, belief in changelings. This involves ill-defined 'spirits', fairies or dwarfs, stealing children away and leaving their own in their place. The child that they leave behind has different names in different countries, but it usually contains some reference to the substitution process that accounts for its presence among humans: *enfant changé* ('changed child') or *changelin* ('changeling') in France, 'changeling' and also 'fairy-child' in England, *Wechselbalg* in Germany.

According to recent evidence,[18] a child is most likely to be taken in the hours and days immediately following its birth, while the child is unbaptised and still does not have a name. It is important not to leave the child unattended during this 'marginal' period; in fact, the child must be hedged around with a whole series of precautions. The door to its room must be carefully closed; a bird or a dog must be left to watch over it; when its parents go out to the fields they must take it with them in its cradle; a candle must be left burning in its room, some salt must be placed near its cradle, etc. It is also recommended that until the child is baptised a flame should be passed around its head each night and morning, or else that it should be swung around the hearth several times. In Scotland, as soon as the child was born and the nurses had given it its first clothes, they would turn it three times round in their arms and bless it and 'shake it upside down three times' to ward off fairies and changelings.[19]

But however many precautions are taken, it sometimes happens that a child is taken and a changeling substituted for it. The child may fall ill and although it always seems hungry, it is never satisfied, and may pine away, leaving one in no doubt that substitution has occurred.

There are ways, however, of getting rid of a changeling once it has been recognised as such, and of recovering the real child. One good method is to make the changeling suffer, so that its true parents will hear its cries of unhappiness and be moved to reclaim it. To achieve this end, one may either beat it or pretend to burn or scald it. Often the changeling is left at a lonely crossroads, or at the point of convergence of three districts, or at the confluence of three rivers. The mother abandons it there and goes away, keeping completely silent, and then returns when the child starts to cry, hoping that her own child will have been replaced and the changeling reclaimed.

Here again recent folklore provides more evidence than past centuries do. In the medieval documents it is always easy to separate belief in changelings, which presupposes substitution, from belief in 'lamias' or vampires, which steal children away, sometimes eating them, but fail to leave another in their place. Stephen of Bourbon writes most of these. The earliest evidence is not always totally clear, however: Notker (d. 1022), in his commentary on Psalm 18 (17), 44, follows custom by translating the expression *filii alieni* ('the sons of strangers', as opposed to Jews) by the German *fremedin chiunt* (*fremde Kinder*), but in the commentary uses the word *wihselinc*, which seems to refer to the notion of substitution (whence the modern German, *Wechselbalg*, a changeling). About 1215, Erike von Repkow talks in the *Mirror of the Saxons*, while referring to deformed or abnormal children, of an *altvil*, a word which has been said to designate changelings.[20] In the same period, Jacques de Vitry quotes the French word *chamium* (from *cambiatus*: 'changed', 'changeling'), but the definition he gives of it is less satisfactory than the name itself, as it takes no account of the phenomenon of substitution which is implicit in the etymology. He says it means 'a child who exhausts the milk of several wetnurses, but to no avail, for it does not grow, and its stomach remains hard and distended. Its body does not grow.'[21] This evidence simply concerns the criteria for recognising changelings. The attitude of the Bishop of Paris, William of Auvergne, in about 1230, is much more precise, and he must have been treated as an authority on the subject, as his opinion is echoed two centuries later by Nicolas of Jawor in his *Treatise of Superstitions* (1405) and by the anonymous author of a *Treatise on Demons* (1415).[22] This is a different context, entailing theological discussions about the nature of demons, and these writers are not therefore concerned (as Jacques de Vitry was) with popular belief in changelings, but with knowing whether demons could engender and thus, where necessary, exchange their children for those of men. According to Nicolas of Jawor (or Jauer), who was Professor at the University of Prague, and later at Heidelberg (he died in 1435), it is the ordinary people who use the argument that there are such things as changelings to assert that incubus demons can engender:

> It is claimed, and generally believed among the people, that incubus demons substitute their own children for human children, and that the women bring them up as if they were their own. This is why they are called 'changelings' (*cambiones*), 'changed' (*cambiati*) or 'exchanged' (*mutati*), substituted for children born of women, put in their place (*suppositi*). They are said to be thin, always crying and unhappy, and so thirsty for milk that no quantity, no matter how abundant, could ever satisfy even one of them.

Nicolas of Jawor clearly deems changelings to exist, but he does not accept that they are, as is popularly supposed, the children of incubus demons; in fact they are the demons themselves, who sometimes assume the form of starving babies, sometimes that of wicked fairies who steal nurslings from their cradles.[23]

Thirteenth-century scholars were much preoccupied with the supposed capacity of incubus demons to procreate. At the beginning of the century, Caesar of Heisterbach recounts the tradition according to which the Huns were descended from the sons of women rejected by the Goths because of their ugliness, and subsequently impregnated by incubus demons in the forest. He recalls that Merlin too was the son of an incubus and a nun.[24] But he also insists that the children of such a union are 'human in nature', not demonic, because in order to impregnate women the demons must use human semen. Shortly after this, the great theologians, Saint Thomas Aquinas and Saint Bonaventura, prove definitively that incubi cannot really procreate; they are simply the vehicles of the human sperm that they have first collected as succubi.[25]

When, therefore, Stephen of Bourbon recounts the evidence of the women he interrogates he specifically says that it is they who say (*quem eorum dicebant*) that the changelings are the fauns' sons. He himself cannot hold such an opinion. But it was a widespread belief that lasted a long time, among the ordinary people at any rate. Changelings, in other words, represent a frightening intrusion by the demonic into everyday life. The word itself, in fact, conjures up all the powers of the devil, so much so that in the fifteenth century to accuse somebody of being a changeling was a terrible insult.[26]

Paradoxically, the wave of witch persecution that raged in Europe between the fifteenth and seventeenth centuries provides no new evidence about changelings. But the explanation for this is simply that the judges' attention was concentrated more on the crimes of the witches themselves, who were accused of taking away children at night and eating them, than on the direct activity of demons.[27]

Martin Luther provides the most valuable information from this period. In his *Table Talk* he comes to the conclusion, on the basis of evidence that he has himself collected, that changelings (*Wechselbalge*) are spirits of water, or the forest, or the underground world; but that in every case they are demons, and evidence of the power of Satan. Luther cites several instances of mothers who have realised that their true child has disappeared, and, when they despair of ever being able to satisfy its appetite, that they have a changeling in their arms.[28]

There are at least three cases where medieval hagiography and its inconographic representations also provide valuable information about changelings.[29]

According to the fourteenth-century *Gesta Romanorum*, the future Saint Lawrence was stolen away soon after birth by the devil, who assumed the form of a new-born child and took his place in the cradle. As is commonly the case at the end of the Middle Ages, the changeling (the word is not in fact used) is the devil in person, not the son of an incubus demon. As for the real child, the devil hung him in a tree in the forest (*silva*), where Pope Sixtus II found him and baptised him, giving him the name of Lawrence. Later the saint returned to his parents and freed them from the little demon, who had, so the narrative has it, been constantly offensive, troublesome and disobedient.[30]

The legend of Saint Bartholomew is almost identical. Like Saint Lawrence, he was the son of a royal couple who had long been barren. They promised God that they would undergo conversion in exchange for the child that they so ardently desired. The devil, afraid of his future enemy, took the new-born infant and abandoned him on a rock, where he was found and taken in by a traveller. He was brought up in a distant land, as a Christian, and at a later date returned to show up the changeling, who (according to a fifteenth-century altarpiece in Tarragona cathedral which has a legend accompanying the picture) had caused four nurses to die of exhaustion in the space of twenty-four years, but to no avail, for he had not grown at all. A manuscript written in Flemish in Brussels has it that the little demon, 'black as pitch, refused to grow and cried in its cradle night and day'. After the three years the priest who, according to this version, rescued Bartholomew, forced him to admit his devilish nature and to flee. Restored to his parents, Bartholomew heard Christ preach and, after their death, he followed him.

There is a painting in the Städel Museum in Frankfurt, called *The Life of Saint Stephen*, which was probably painted by the Sienese Martino di Bartolomeo (1389–1434), and this too represents a changeling who is constantly famished and yet 'does not grow at all' (see Illustration 3). The principal hagiographic narrative about the protomartyr, whose feast day is 26 December, is of course contained in the Acts of the Apostles, chapters 6 and 7, and there is obviously no mention of a changeling there! Nonetheless, the cult of Saint Stephen gave rise to a *Vita fabulosa*, quite different from apostolic tradition, the oldest manuscript version of which dates from the tenth or eleventh century.[31] The childhood of Saint Stephen, which is not mentioned at all in Acts, is described in detail in the *Life*. According to this text, when Stephen was born, Satan, 'in the shape of a man', got into his parents' house, went up to the cradle, stole the child and left a statuette (*idolum*) in his place. Having then taken the baby across the sea, Satan left him outside the door of a bishop called Julian. There he was suckled by a white doe which addressed the bishop, when he opened the door, with the following words: 'Here is the man that God has sent you!' Stephen was brought up by the bishop, became a wise *juvenis*, started preaching in Asia, and performed his first miracle by raising someone from the dead.

Then he returned to the city of Galilee, and to his parents, where he

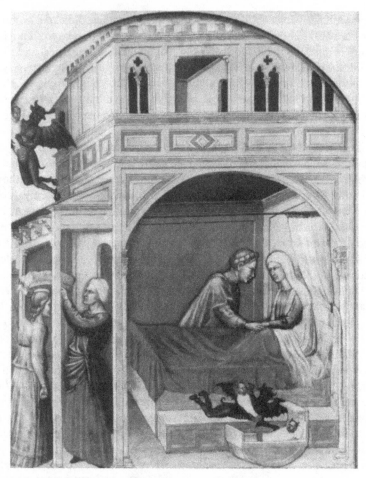

3 *Life of Saint Stephen*, by Martino di Bartolomeo, Siena (1389–1434).
(a) The devil substitutes a changeling for the child.

ordered the 'demon' to declare 'whose son he was'. Although dumb up to
then, it replied 'Do not kill me, Stephen, and I shall rejoin all those who are
your enemies.' The saint's refusal provoked 'Satan' into 'hissing, bellowing
like a bull, and every kind of animal noise'. Then Stephen said to his father:
'I am your son whom Satan took from the cradle and replaced with his own
son (*suum genitum*).'

It is clearly a changeling that is being described here, even if there is no
specific name given to the diabolic being who was exchanged for the child.
But this text does seem rather hesitant as to the nature of the 'idol', which
appears to be inanimate up until the moment at which the saint forces it to
speak and to reveal that it is the son of the devil. This impression is

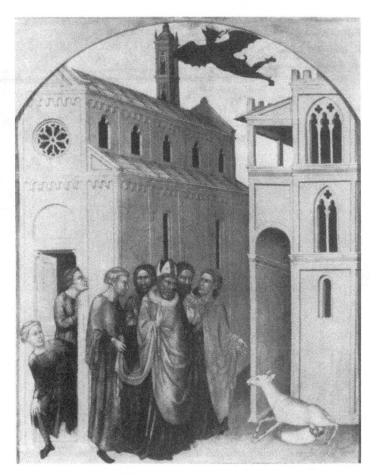

(b) A white doe suckles the child, and the bishop receives it.

reinforced by Martino di Bartolomeo's painting, in which the changeling, wrapped in swaddling-clothes, looks just like a wooden statue (but then so does the actual baby that is being carried into the air by a winged devil)! However, the painting is more than just an illustration of the text. The episodes where the child is stolen, and where he is suckled by the doe, are faithful to the written text, but when the saint returns, not content with unmasking the demon, he has him consigned to the flames. This variant is not mentioned in either of the two known manuscripts of the *Vita fabulosa*, and may perhaps stem from an oral tradition. What is interesting about this pictorial version is, therefore, its fidelity to folk beliefs. The people who looked at the picture would automatically have assumed that the baby

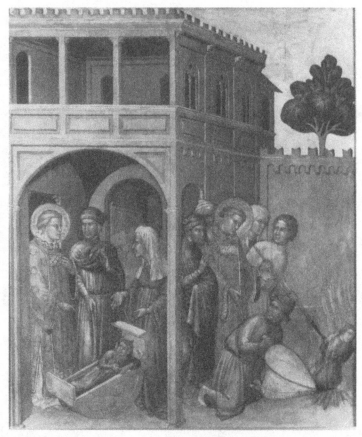

(c) Saint Stephen, having returned to his parents, discovers the changeling and has him thrown into the flames.

thrown into the fire was a changeling, because it had not grown since the first episode, whereas Saint Stephen was by that time a young man.

The fact that the saint returns, and unmasks the changeling who took his place at birth, gives the hagiographic narrative a miraculous dimension which is in striking contrast to the exigencies of the folk rite. Of all the documents in the medieval period touching upon the subject of changelings, Stephen of Bourbon's *exemplum* would therefore seem, on account of its early date and the wealth of information it contains, to be one of the best sources of evidence. It is true that the name 'changeling' is not applied to the sick children that the mothers try to give back to the fauns. But the substitution that had taken place is described fully, and for the first time the rite designed to achieve the reverse exchange and to allow the women to recover their own children is described in all its detail.

The aim of the rite's third sequence seems to be to test the efficacity of the previous sequence. If the child can resist the cold of the river, it is taken as a proof that he is the woman's true child, given back by the fauns. A changeling, on the other hand, is too feeble to survive this treatment, and if he dies at once or soon afterwards this is because the fauns have not agreed to take him back. This form of trial by water may be compared with one of the forms of ordeal, the aim of which was not to find the culprit but to confirm or deny the guilt of the person accused, according as to whether they sank or swam when ducked publicly in cold water. This old Germanic practice (the word 'ordeal' means 'judgement', *Urtheil*) was used in the guise of the 'judgement of God' until the modern period as a means of identifying witches both male and female.[32] However, it is important not to underestimate the differences, both formal and functional, between the two practices. What they have in common is the same 'all or nothing' logic. In the 'judgement of God' the accused is innocent if he sinks and proclaimed a witch if he swims; here, if the child survives he is really a human child, and if he dies he is a demon. The same bald logic is to be found in many other folk rituals. In Scotland, when a child was brought home from church after being baptised a woman would swing him gently three or four times over a flame, saying 'May the flames consume you now or never.'[33] The rite of passage concentrates the child's whole destiny within the one moment; the baptismal water has given him eternal life and the fire of the flame symbolises the hell fire that will never be able to claim him if it does not do so at this instant. The opposition between the symbols of fire and water, in this baptismal rite as in the one in the *exemplum*, represents the basic dualism of the forces at stake: life and death, men and demons.

The relations between our rite and baptism can be set out in more detail. As we have seen, it is baptism that offers the best form of protection against changelings. Being a Christian is a defence against the attacks of the demon, even though it is not sufficient to keep him away forever. The same symbolic elements are found in both rites, namely, salt, fire and water. The triple immersion of the baptismal child 'in the name of the Father, the Son and the Holy Ghost', that was still used in the thirteenth century,[34] corresponds, multiplied by three, to the number of immersions in the Chalaronne. Yet there is no mention of baptism, either in the legend and its parallel versions or in the rite. But it is clear enough why this should be the case, for the children involved have already been baptised. Traditionally the clergy waited for Easter eve and then baptised all the babies in the community at once. But it became increasingly common in the twelfth and thirteenth centuries to administer baptism as quickly as possible after birth, or at least in the days immediately following, in order to lower the risk of children dying without being baptised. Baptism ensured a child's salvation if he died soon after being born, which happened in one case out of every two or three.

It also exorcised diabolic forces, drove away evil spirits and, if the child survived, made him well developed, good-looking and prevented him from being drowned or being eaten by wolves.[35] More particularly, baptism was thought to turn a new-born babe into a 'little human'.[36] There is no doubt the knight's son saved by the greyhound has this 'little human' quality, as do the children saved from the fauns. The rite of substitution must not be confused with baptism. But although they are very similar in some respects, the function of the former may perhaps have been to reawaken the effects of baptism in those exceptional cases in which it had turned out to have been incapable of keeping children safe from the clutches of illness and demons.

This rite must clearly have caused the deaths of a fair number of children. Brought there in the first place because they were sickly or ill, they were left naked in the wood and then ducked nine times in the cold water of the river. They were also subjected to the dangers from fire and wolves during this temporary exposure. How could children in that condition survive such treatment? When Stephen of Bourbon accused the mothers of infanticide, he cannot have been too far from the truth. But we need also to take into account the implications of belief in changelings. The children who died were *not* the children of these mothers, they were the children of devils. If the rite had a function it was to select or, in the fullest sense of the term, to recognise the real children. It was thus a rite of rebirth, identification and admission. The mothers did not regard it as ritualised infanticide, for the children who died were not born of human beings, but as a rite whose purpose was to identify their real children and save them.

One of the mothers, however, instead of allowing the implacable logic of the rite to continue to its fatal conclusion, retraced her steps in order to chase off the wolf that was about to devour 'her' child. But if the wolf was about to devour it, must it not have been a changeling? This clearly illustrates both the threefold function of belief in changelings and its limits and contradictions. First, it was a means of explaining sickness or abormality. Secondly, it allowed parents to suppress social reality and the burden involved in raising a sick child, not by curing the illness, but by changing the identity of the sick child; once he had become the devil's child he could be removed with impunity from the human collectivity. Thirdly, in a period in which the increasingly prevalent practice of annual confession was deepening individual conscience and developing the notion of guilt, this belief provided a means for mothers to avoid reproaching themselves for the death of their children. This explains the paradoxical nature of the rite, and also, no doubt, Stephen of Bourbon's difficulty in understanding the real reasons for its existence. The mothers certainly felt it to be a life-saving rite for their children, when in fact it ended up by killing the weakest of them. But if these children were doomed anyway, the cult of Saint Guinefort probably did little to alter the demographic curve of this peasant community.

6

THE UNITY OF THE NARRATIVE

The peasants interrogated by Stephen of Bourbon were aware of the indissoluble link between the legend and the rite, for they introduced the legend as a narrative of the origins of the cult. I shall not adopt this explanation, nor shall I try to present the rite as the enactment of the legend. But legend and rite are nevertheless inseparable, for their themes overlap and, more important still, they are united by the logical development of a single narrative.

The legend, like the rite, displays some anxiety as to the safety of children under severe threat. This may seem a somewhat surprising assertion, given that, according to Philippe Ariès, the 'idea of childhood' did not exist in the Middle Ages, and young children were not put into any precise category, which is why the terminology is so vague. At the very most there is a 'superficial idea of childhood', which was sometimes applied to one of the rare children who survived; this came into its own at the beginning of the modern period, in the seventeenth century, and Ariès calls it 'coddling' – the child is seen as 'an amusing little thing' and 'we play with him as if he was a little animal, a shameless little monkey. . .'. The idea of childhood finally emerged in a more recent period, along with the strengthening of the bourgeois family unit and with schooling, which delayed the child's entry into the adult world, and thus encouraged society to grant him a real status.

Philippe Ariès's thesis, which was first put forward in 1960, was corroborated some four years later, at least as far as the medieval period was concerned, by Jacques Le Goff, who wrote: 'It has been said that there are no children in the Middle Ages, and that there are only young adults.'[1]

But more recently, through analysing documentary evidence and a social milieu that closely resemble the ones in question here, Le Roy Ladurie has challenged Ariès's conclusions. In the upper Ariège, in the first half of the fourteenth century, the lady of Châteauverdun was reluctant to leave her child, still in the cradle, to go and join the heretics:

> She wanted to see it before leaving. When she saw it she kissed it; then the child began to laugh. She had started to go out of the room where the infant lay so she came back to it again. The child began to laugh again; and so on, several times, so that she couldn't bear to tear herself away from the child. Seeing this she said to her maidservant: 'Take him out of the house!'

One might suppose that this was an exclusively aristocratic attitude, but such is not the case, for similar attitudes are found among simple peasants. Sybille Pierre was unable to bring herself to allow her little Jacotte to die of hunger when she was gravely ill and had received the Cathar *consolamentum*, and ended up disobeying both the Parfait and her husband:

> When my husband and Prades Tavernier had left the house, I could not bear it any longer. I couldn't let my daughter die before my very eyes. So I put her to the breast. . .[2]

These texts do seem to confirm the existence, at two different levels of society, of a medieval idea of childhood. But this narrow and not entirely accurate account of Philippe Ariès's argument does him an injustice. For he does differentiate between the 'affection' that parents, especially mothers, feel for their children, and the 'idea of childhood', given that the category of 'childhood' was only hazily defined in the medieval period. He has also shown that nurslings, constantly vulnerable to death and therefore given particular care and attention, received much more attention than slightly older children, who merged into the adult world. On the other hand, one must agree with Le Roy Ladurie when, following J.-L. Flandrin, he criticises Ariès for having based his researches almost entirely on documents and pictures which express the views of the élite, and ignoring 'the massive, unwritten reality of the affectivity of the lower classes'.

Philippe Ariès's argument is fundamentally correct, but it requires supplementation and qualification. Other kinds of documentary evidence need to be analysed, and the book's thesis needs to be qualified along the lines already indicated by the author elsewhere, and which have since been specified by researchers working on related topics.[3] Childhood does not constitute a well-defined category in the Middle Ages; but an emerging awareness of childhood and children can be detected in the medieval period, given certain conditions.

The folk culture provides one of the conditions for the emerging awareness of the medieval child. As the documents that deal with the Pyrenean village of Montaillou at the beginning of the fourteenth century show, along with Stephen of Bourbon's *exemplum* half a century earlier (or, indeed, a comparable twelfth-century text by Gervase of Tilbury),[4] the child in folklore breaks through the silence of the texts and makes his presence felt. He grizzles, he fidgets, he is rocked, cared for, suckled and loved. He is, in short, acknowledged.

There are three reasons for this. Even though the documents that contain information about folk culture in the Middle Ages are written by clerics, they are not designed to improve the intellectual classifications of the Ages of Life, nor are they meant to enclose the course of earthly existence within the theological perspective that the promise of an after-life and of salvation implies. These documents frequently articulate the preoccupations of lay people, and reveal their familial and lineal concerns. For them, the child is the future inheritor who must be protected from the ever-present threat of death, so as to ensure the continuity of the lineage and the survival of the chivalric estate or of the peasant 'house'. For the church, on the other hand, the child could well be an obstacle to salvation, in that its parents' generosity might be focussed upon it. Whatever they had given as alms to the poor (and to the church!) before the child's birth would now be jealously guarded, so as to increase its heritage; and whatever time they had used to spend on their own salvation would now be given up to looking after the baby.[5]

There is another reason why the documents concerned with folk culture should become increasingly aware of children, namely that they devote a lot of space to the supernatural, whether the authors are denouncing demons and witches, or whether they are fascinated by the marvels recounted by oral tradition.

The medieval child, a 'changeful'[6] being, who therefore worries and confuses adults by an ambivalence which cannot be pinned down or classified, attracts the supernatural. He attracts it in an ambiguous fashion appropriate to his 'diversity': on the positive side, he is the child of miracles and hagiography; on the negative side, he is the child of the devil, or sometimes the accomplice, but more commonly the victim, of a witch. The second part of the *exemplum* treats the child from this angle.

There is a third and final reason for the child's pivotal role in folklore. In documents that often shed some light on family or kinship matters, the child is always part of a family, never alone. And here the attention paid to the child appears, from the Middle Ages onwards, to be one aspect of the slow rise of the restricted family unit. Religious iconography provides evidence for this, in that the child who begins as a scaled-down version of an adult, as nothing more than a hieratic piece of wood or stone in the lap of a Romanesque Virgin, becomes more childlike in the Gothic period, and at the same time acquires a mother, a grandmother, a father, and, before too long, cousins. The *exemplum* is open to a similar interpretation, for the first part contains a representation of the model chivalric family, such as the peasants whose confessions Stephen of Bourbon heard must have imagined it from the outside. This model is an abstraction from the vast network of family relationships that George Duby has found in noble genealogies and charters, and entails a reduction of such a network to its simplest form, namely, father, mother, and nurse, with the male child as focus. (As I have emphasised, the nurse is an outward sign of nobility.) There are no nurses, however, in the description of the peasant rite. No father, either, in fact, but just the mother on her own with her child, and an old woman who knows the gestures and the words that can cure it. So it is that, on the margins of the inhabited areas, women and children confront illness and fate on their own.

In fact, as both legend and rite make plain, the child is in grave danger. The snake in the legend is hardly described at all. Indeed, we cannot assume that it comes out of the castle wall, as it does in most of the parallel narratives. But the 'outside', whence it comes, appears all the more threatening for being so ill defined. In the context of the cult site, this 'outside' is clearly the *silva*, the forest that is the abode of wolves and fauns. In the legend the snake is not explicitly called 'Satan', but its great size (*maximus*) indicates as much. It is closely associated, moreover, with the demons, the fauns, and the diabolic wolf mentioned in the description of the rite.

In the legend, the child is saved by the dog which has been left with him. The presence of the dog recalls one of the protective measures customarily taken against changelings, in which an animal, generally a dog, is left near the cradle. The same thing occurs in N7, which is the only version of the narrative in which the nurses take the precaution of taking the cradle with them and leaving it at the foot of the wall, instead of leaving it in the empty house. But this precaution is, of course, inadequate!

Above all else, the legend and the rite are united by a series of logical relationships. The murder of the greyhound that saved the child sanctions his veneration as a martyr and saviour of children. Planting trees by the well where the greyhound's body was buried preserves the 'memory of the deed' and initiates the wooded place where the rite occurs. The depopulation of the estate 'by its inhabitants' allows the subsequent return of peasants drawn there by the oral tradition (*audientes*).

Thus the whole of the narrative describes a dual diachronic transformation, of the status of the greyhound on the one hand, and of the appearance of the countryside on the other. The greyhound, the knight's faithful companion, is unjustly killed; he is dead, but buried in such a way as to preserve the memory of what he has done; his death makes him a martyr, and it is not long before he is honoured under the name of Saint Guinefort. Parallel to this set of events, we find the *castrum* where the knight and his family live; after the murder of the greyhound it is destroyed 'by divine will' and the estate becomes a desert; it is not long before the peasants come to the area and make it an object of pilgrimage. But the crucial thing is that the site has meanwhile acquired a new purpose and new users. From being the house of a *miles* – the representative of the ruling, warrior class – it becomes a religious *locus*, visited by those who were ruled, the *rustici*. I shall now present an interim schematisation of this threefold alteration, for the problems that it raises are at the heart of the historical interpretation of the whole of the document.

Table 3 *Transformation in the course of the narrative*

	I	2	3
Status of the greyhound	domestic animal	thought to be a wild beast, and therefore killed	saint and martyr called Guinefort
Appearance of the countryside	seigneurial *castrum*	destroyed and uninhabited (but trees growing)	*locus* of pilgrimage
Actors	the *miles* and his family	no inhabitants any longer	the *rustici* come on pilgrimage

PART 3

Saint Guinefort

7

THE OTHER CULT SITES

The peasants of the Dombes gave the dog in the legend the name of Saint Guinefort, martyr. Stephen of Bourbon's astonishment at hearing this saint's name for the first time might lead one to think that they had invented it themselves. But such was not the case, for since the eleventh century at least, Saint Guinefort, martyr, had been revered in many other places, but in a human form.

The *Life* of Saint Guinefort (*Guinifortus, Gunifortus*) would seem to have been composed between the eighth and the twelfth century. We know it through two manuscripts, a *Passio Sancti Guiniforti*, kept at Latran, and the *Miracula Sancti Guniforti*, of the fourteenth century, kept at Novare. Besides a narrative of the saint's life, the latter gives us a list of miracles from which several of his adepts must have benefited during the first half of the fourteenth century.[1]

Saint Guinefort is said to have lived at the time of the Emperors Diocletian and Maximilian. Fleeing the persecutions directed against the Christians by the 'heretic infidels', he left his native Ireland (*Scotia*) with his brother Guiniboldus and his two sisters. The latter are not mentioned in the *Passio*, but according to the Novare manuscript, they were called Pusillana and Favilla. At the time of the crossing of Germany, they were martyred by the 'Teutonic tribes'. Their feast day is 9 January. Eluding the authorities, the two brothers reached Italy. They began to preach at Como, they were arrested and the local prince had Guniboldus beheaded. But, at night, the Christians made off in secret with his body and buried it. His feast day is 14 October.

Guinefort continued his journey alone, and, at Milan, started preaching again. The 'tyrant' condemned him to be beheaded outside the town. As he was taken out to be executed, his executioners stoned him, pierced him with arrows and beat him with iron rods. Reckoning that he would not survive up to the hour appointed for his execution, they 'so filled the holy martyr with arrows that he resembled a hedgehog'. When he fell to the ground, they believed him to be dead and abandoned him.

His body bristling with arrows, but still alive, Guinefort dragged himself as far as Pavia, where a Christian took him into his home, close to the church of Santa Romana. The *Passio* also states that numerous blind persons, invalids and lepers were miraculously cured there. The saint's feast day at Pavia is 22 August, which is the day upon which he was buried.

This hagiographic legend closely resembles that of Saint Sebastian, whose cult is also closely tied to the city of Pavia. Martyred at Rome by Diocletian, Sebastian, so *The Golden Legend* has it, was also so pierced by arrows that he resembled a hedgehog. But he survived this execution; his executioners, believing him to be dead, abandoned him. Once recovered he sought out the Emperor and reproached him for persecuting the Christians. This time he was whipped to death and his body was thrown into a privy. But the saint appeared to Saint Lucina and revealed to her where his body was. She set out to find it and buried it with dignity near the bodies of the apostles. Saint Sebastian's feast day is 20 January.

During July, August and September 680, the plague raged in Pavia. It was revealed to someone that the epidemic would cease if an altar to Saint Sebastian were raised in the basilica of San Pietro-in-Vincoli. Relics were brought from Rome to Pavia and the plague did immediately cease.[2]

Saint Sebastian's reputation as protector against the plague (the martyr's arrows were compared to attacks of the illness) flourished, particularly after the return of the plague to the West in 1348. Saint Sebastian shared his title as anti-plague saint with several others, namely the Virgin Mary, Saint Roch, Saint Anthony, and with dozens of other 'minor'[3] saints as well. At Pavia, Saint Guinefort was numbered among them.

Saint Guinefort's cult seems to have remained quiescent at Pavia until the middle of the fourteenth century.[4] An account of an episcopal visit in 1236 mentions the presence of the saint's body in the church of Santa Maria, near to San Romagna, and a chapel is mentioned after 1330. The cult would actually seem to have gained in intensity during the fourteenth century, owing to the interest shown in it by the patrician Morzano family. This family was certainly not unfamiliar with the composition of Saint Guinefort's *Miracles*. Thus, the saint is said to have pacified the divine wrath which fell upon the Morzanos when one of them had committed a sacrilege. The crucifix of the saint's chapel having, in falling, wounded his wife, he had thrown it into the river! But, following this sacrilege, his lineage was so decimated that finally, yielding to the Morzanos' prayers, Saint Guinefort interceded on their behalf with God, and obtained his pardon. Another miracle also concerned a child of this family, one Albricus de Morzano, lame from birth, who was cured in this saint's tomb when five years old, in the presence of a large number of his relatives, men and women, who had come to celebrate the feast of Saint Guinefort.

But there are other miracles which indicate that Saint Guinefort's fame had already spread even further. Thus, at Milan, the saint's appearance served to establish the innocence of a knight of Como and his servant, who had been wrongfully accused of theft. In 1340, a merchant from Genoa, who had accidentally fallen into the sea at Péra (Constantinople), had just enough time to invoke Saint Guinefort (*O Sancte Guniforte, adjuva me!*), whereupon he immediately appeared above the church of Saint Michael and saved him from drowning by pulling him out by his hair. In 1350, when the Black Death was raging, a child by the name of Todescus, having fallen ill, was saved from death when his brother Franciscus invoked Saint Guinefort. Three years later, as a token of his gratitude, Franciscus had the door and bell of the church refurbished. In 1356, he revisited this church and testified to the authenticity of this miracle.

In the middle of the fourteenth century, as is clear from the above accounts, Saint Guinefort did not yet specialise in a particular type of miracle. But he had already gained a certain fame as a saint who was capable of keeping the plague at bay. When a new wave of the epidemic occurred, in 1374, he acquired the reputation of being a specialist. It was at this date that the members of a brotherhood for which we have records from the beginning of the thirteenth century took the name of 'Disciplinati di S. Guniforto', based themselves around this church and invoked him, particularly as a defence against the plague. It is also from this period onwards that the saint comes to be represented as a knight (*miles, cavaliere*), in the manner of Saint Sebastian, even though there is nothing in his *Life* to justify such an identification. Finally, in litanies, he is now associated with the great saints who give protection against the plague, i.e., Saint Sebastian, Saint Roch, Saint Christopher.

In the fifteenth century there were yet other factors encouraging the growth of the cult, such as the Visconti's generosity, the official adoption by the Faculty of Jurists of Saint Guinefort's patronage in 1415, and, in 1419, the granting of indulgences to the pilgrims of Saint Guinefort by Pope Martin V. The Christian name *Guniforto* seems to have been fairly common at this period in Pavia, and the cult also expanded outside that town. Thus, in 1446, a chapel of Saints James and Guinefort is mentioned in the church of San Lorenzo at Milan, beside the gate of Pavia (*Porta ticinensis*).

The cult was still thriving in Pavia after the medieval period. In January 1650, the regular canonesses of the Monasterio Nuovo won the right to transfer the saint's body to their own church. A veritable archaeological excavation took place under the altar of the chapel of Saint Guinefort, and the body was recovered at the end of three days. Some relics were disinterred and distributed, and the saint's remains were taken to the sisters' establishment in a procession. Further relics were removed in 1670 and 1726, in order to 'strengthen the cult of Saint Guinefort' by spreading his precious remains far and wide. In 1768, the suppression of the monastery resulted in a fourth dispersal, with what remained of the body being transferred to the parish church of S. Maria Gualteri. Upon this occasion the saint was dressed as a Roman soldier, helmeted, with his martyr's palm in his hand, and stretched out upon a red piece of damask fringed with gold,

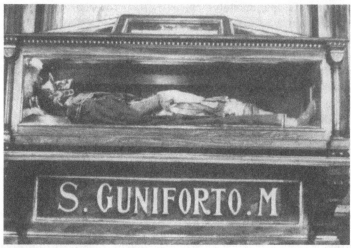

4 Saint Guinefort of Pavia
  (a) The shrine

and thus displayed in an imposing, gilded shrine, for the veneration of the faithful. This is how Saint Guinefort still appears today in the chapel of the Church of Saints Gervase and Protase (see Illustration 4), where he was taken in 1790, as if he were a Roman soldier, but in the Gothic style, and reduced by a succession of removals of relics to the dimensions of a big and somewhat ridiculous doll. Apart from the skull, nothing of the original body would seem to be present in this mannequin. There is a small reliquary beside the head, which contains some fragments of bone (cf. Illustration 4b). Under the altar is kept a casket which bears the inscription 'S. Guiniboldo', and which is thought to contain relics of Saint Guinefort's brother.

The successive removal of relics must clearly have helped to spread the cult of Saint Guinefort (Map 1: nos 8 to 15). Thus, those relics that were removed in 1670 enabled the new church of Casatisma, in the diocese of Tortona, to be dedicated to Saint Guinefort. In 1726, the church of Nosate, close to Milan, also received the name and a few fragments of the saint. In 1769, several parishes in Milan were also so honoured, and in 1896 the Bishop of Pavia actually offered a Norman curé a relic for his parish.[5]

Meanwhile, in Pavia, the cult had not fallen into decline. The parish and episcopal authorities encouraged it, as Canon Moiraghi's little pamphlet, published in 1916 with the bishop's *imprimatur*, shows. It contains a summary of the saint's life, recalls the many favours that his devotees have been granted, and implies that it is particularly fitting to invoke him for the cure of sick children. In the second half of this little work, it is no longer a

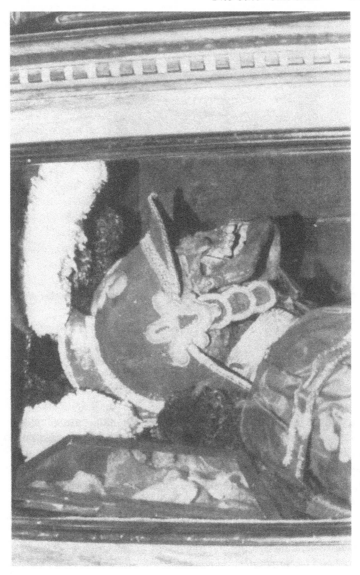

(b) Detail of the head

question of bodily sufferings, but of the faith and love of God, which the saint is empowered to strengthen in those of the faithful who pray to him.[6]

More recently still, in 1966, on the occasion of the patron saints' day of 11 September the parish newsletter of the Church of Saints Gervase and Protase reminded the faithful of the life of Saint Guinefort, 'missionary',

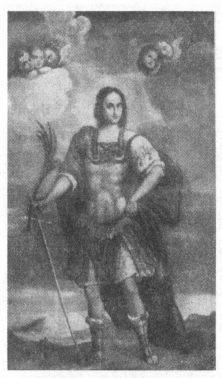

(c) A pious picture, collected by the author in 1976.

and praised his talents as a healer, 'especially in the case of children'.[7] The article is followed by a statement from the priest, who castigates those who hesitate before calling a priest to the bedside of the sick, but adds: 'I take pleasure in the great number of people, a number indeed far greater than one might suppose, who invoke Saint Guinefort on behalf of the sick and dying'. In the church, in front of the shrine, holy images are placed at the disposal of the faithful; they represent the saint dressed as a Roman soldier, his sword and martyr's palm in his right hand. The other side features the text of a prayer which one is supposed to address to the saint. It praises his courage as missionary and martyr and begs Saint Guinefort to revive the faith and to relieve the sufferings of the faithful. A hundred days' indulgence is promised to whoever recites this prayer.

The cult of Saint Guinefort at Pavia clearly no longer enjoys the glory of centuries past. Nevertheless, in the old quarter surrounding the church of Saints Cosmas and Damian, those attached to traditional forms of worship are still very devoted to Saint Guinefort. There are, moreover, obvious discrepancies between these forms of worship and the cult such as it is defined in official documents, but the local clergy would seem to have come to terms with them. Thus, in 1854, an old priest from Nosate gave his own version of the saint's life: 'He must have been one of our Lombards, who fought beneath the gates of Milan, in the days of Gregory VII. He was killed there and his body has been preserved in the church of Saints Gervase and Protase at Pavia.' A proverb, still current in Pavia, illustrates the alternative faced by those sick persons who devoted themselves to him:

> Chi si vota a S. Boniforto
> Dopo tre giorni è vivo o morto.[8]

The saint was most commonly invoked by those who were dying, and who hoped for a rapid and complete recovery, unless death, precipitated by the invocation itself, were to intervene. But, in the opinion of the present incumbent of the church (October 1976), there are yet other reasons for invoking him. Thus, a 'witch' who lives close to the Piazza della Vittoria, but whom I did not succeed in tracing, advises young women in search of a husband to go and pray to the saint. And recently, some workers threatened with redundancy prayed to the saint, successfully it would seem, to keep them in work, whereupon they arranged to have a thanksgiving mass said in his honour.

Are Saint Guinefort (*Guinifortus*), of whom we have evidence at Pavia, at least since 1236 (the first definite date, but the *Passio* is even earlier), and Saint *Guinefortis*, venerated by the peasants of the Dombes around 1250, one and the same?

One is a man, and the other a dog. But their names are similar, and both are called 'saints' and, more precisely, 'martyrs'. Their respective legends are, however, utterly different. Thus, the one from Pavia contains no reference to a dog, not even a peripheral one. There is only one point of comparison: one was condemned to be beheaded (and was finally pierced with arrows), the other was actually killed with a sword (but N1 does not specify if he was beheaded).

The actual cults would seem to have more in common. Both cure the sick, and children in particular, and both save people in situations of extreme danger. One can thus compare the formula from Pavia ('Whoever devotes himself to Saint Bonifort/Will, within three days, be living or dead') with the final sequence of the peasant rite from the Dombes, in that the child who is immersed in the river either dies immediately or is definitively saved.

Finally, it is worth noting the coincidence in chronology, namely, that both cults are first cited around the middle of the thirteenth century.

There is thus no clearly observable relation between them, and yet it is worth clinging to the hypothesis that such a relation does indeed exist. If, moreover, one takes into account the geographical and historical diffusion of the cult at Pavia, this hypothesis seems quite a probable one.

In 1082, a charter at the Abbey of Cluny, in Burgundy, records a

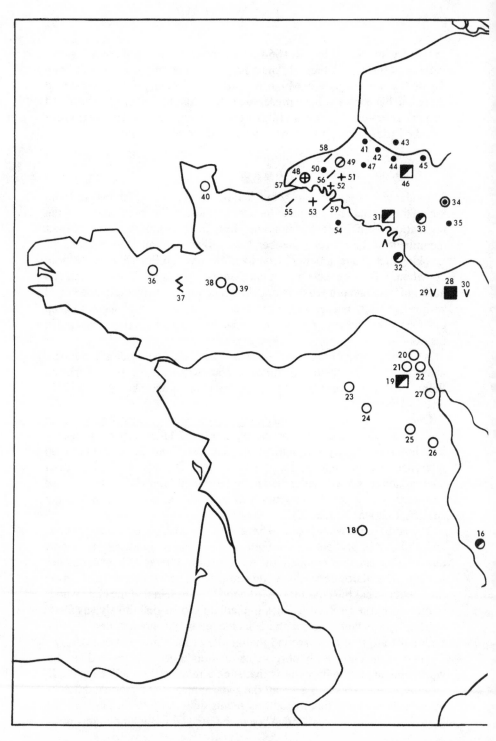

Map 1 The cult of Saint Guinefort, eleventh to twelfth century (Graphics Laboratory of the E.H.E.S.S.)

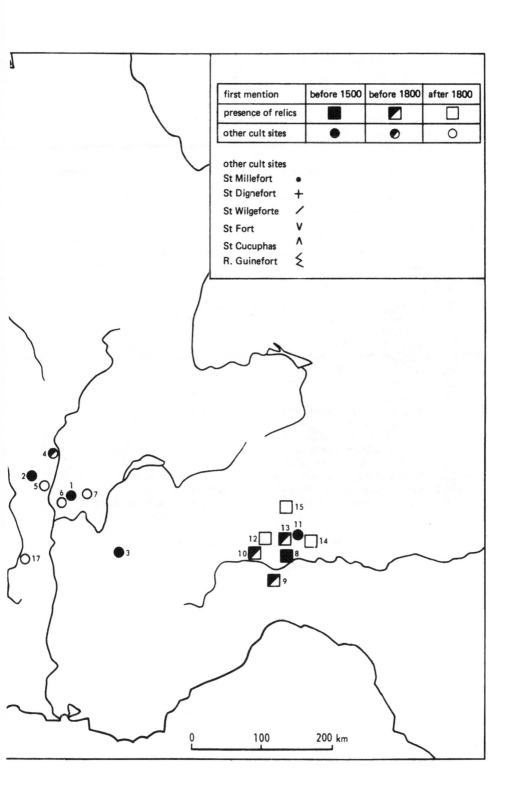

first mention	before 1500	before 1800	after 1800
presence of relics	■	◪	□
other cult sites	●	◕	○

other cult sites
St Millefort   ●
St Dignefort   +
St Wilgeforte   /
St Fort   ∨
St Cucuphas   ∧
R. Guinefort   ⩾

0   100   200 km

MAP 1

List of cult sites

1. Saint Guinefort's wood (Sandrans *commune*, Bourg-en-Bresse *arrondissement*, Ain) (around 1250–1940)
2. Altar at Cluny III (Mâcon *arrondissement*, Saône-et-Loire) (1485, perhaps from 1131 onwards)
3. Allevard (Grenoble *arrondissement*, Isère): 'Saint Guinefort's manse', in a charter at Cluny (1082)
4. Tournus (Saône-et-Loire): 'Mont Saint Guinefort' and hermitage (1647)
5. Crêches (Mâcon *arrondissement*, Saône-et-Loire): invoked at the end of the nineteenth century
6. Béreins (Saint Trivier *commune*, Bourg-en-Bresse *arrondissement*, Ain): castle chapel
7. Marleux (Bourg-en-Bresse *arrondissement*, Ain): Saint Guinefort's cherry-tree
8. Pavia: probably from the eleventh century at least. Church of Saint Gervase and Saint Protais
9. Casatisma (1670)
10. Nosate (1726)
11. Milan: church of Saint Lawrence: chapel of Saint James and Saint Guinefort (1446)
12. Torre d'Isola (1835)
13. Mirabello (before 1854)
14. Villanterio (1827)
15. Vill'Albese (nineteenth century)
16. Le Puy (Upper Loire): chapel of Saint Guinefort (1625)
17. Bords du Lignon
18. Saint Pardoux-Corbier (Brive-la-Gaillarde *arrondissement*, Corrèze)
19. Saint Junien (Upper Vienne): crypt said to be Saint Guinefort's
20. Bourges (Cher) (end of the eleventh century)
21. Saint Satur (Sancerre *arrondissement*, Cher)
22. Méry-ès-Bois (Sancerre *arrondissement*, Cher)
23. La Chapelle d'Anguillon: castle chapel (Sancerre *arrondissement*, Cher)
24. Levroux (Châteauroux *arrondissement*, Indre): collegial
25. Verneuil-sur-Igneraie (La Châtre *arrondissement*, Indre): statue in the church
26. Tortezais (Montluçon *arrondissement*, Allier): the church's patron
27. Valgny-le-Monial (Gannat *arrondissement*, Allier)
28. Sancoins (Saint-Amand-Mont-Rond *arrondissement*, Cher): chapel
29. Sens (Yonne) (from 1241)
30. Malicorne (d'Auxerre *arrondissement*, Yonne)
31. La-Fontaine-Saint-Fort
32. Piscop (Pontoise *arrondissement*, Oise) (at least since 1684)
33. Tigery (d'Evry *arrondissement*, Essonne) (eighteenth-century chapel)
34. Dammartin-en-Goële (Meaux *arrondissement*, Seine-et-Marne) (chapel from the seventeenth century)
35. Bouillant (near Crépy-en-Valois, Senlis *arrondissement*, Oise): statue of Saint Guinefort (or Millefort?)
36. La Ferté-sous-Jouarre (Meaux *arrondissement*, Seine-et-Marne)
37. Lamballe (Saint-Brieue *arrondissement*, Côtes-du-Nord)
38. R. Guinefort (tributary of the Rance)
39. Saint Broladre (Pleine-Fougères canton, Ile-et-Vilaine)
40. Roz-sur-Couesnon (Pleine-Fougères canton, Ile-et-Vilaine)
41. Golleville (Cherbourg *arrondissement*, Manche)
42. La Bouvaque (Somme): chapel of Saint Millefort (from 1419 at least)

43. Saint-Aubin-Rivière (Amiens *arrondissement*, Somme): chapel of Saint Millefort (around 1858)
44. Forest-Montiers (Abbeville *arrondissement*, Somme)
45. Camps-en-Amiénois (Amiens *arrondissement*, Somme): Saint Millefort chapel of Saint Millefort, around 1850
46. La Neuville-sous-Corbie (Amiens *arrondissement*, Somme): lazar-house of Saint Millefort, statue on the altar
47. Montdidier (Somme): Cluniac priory, relics of Saint Guinefort (before 1660)
48. Gorenflos (Abbeville *arrondissement*, Somme); domain said to be that of Saint Millefort
49. Gonfreville-L'Orcher (Le Havre *arrondissement*, Seine-Maritime): priory of Saint Dignefort (1738) or Guinefort
50. Arques (Saint Omer *arrondissement*, Pas-de-Calais): chapel (rebuilt in 1697) of Saint Wilgeforte or Guinefort or Dignefort
51. Blangy (Amiens *arrondissement*, Somme): chapel of Saint Millefort?
52. Saussay-en-Caux (Forges-les-Eaux *canton*, Seine-Maritime): statue of Saint Dignefort
53. Rouen: Carmelite convent (from the fifteenth century): Saint Dignefort, patron of the brotherhood
54. Gruchet-la-Valasse (Le Havre *arrondissement*, Seine-Maritime): statue of Saint Dignefort(?)
55. Appeville (Bernay *arrondissement*, Eure): pilgrimage to Saint Millefort
56. Montpinçon (Saint Pierre-sur-Dives *canton*, Calvados): pilgrimage to Saint Wilgeforte
57. Fauville (Yvetot *arrondissement*, Seine-Maritime): pilgrimage to Saint Wilgeforte
58. Daubeuf-Serville (Le Havre *arrondissement*, Seine-Maritime): pilgrimage to Saint Wilgeforte
59. Vittefleur (Dieppe *arrondissement*, Seine-Maritime): pilgrimage to Saint Wilgeforte
60. Flamanville (Rouen *arrondissement*, Seine-Maritime): pilgrimage to Saint Wilgeforte

donation that was made to the monks of a messuage of Saint Guinifortus (*mansus sancti Guiniforti cum omni possessione sua*) situated in the neighbourhood of Allevard, now in the *département* of Isère.[9] I would simply note the early date of this text, and the spelling of the saint's name, which is identical to that of the *Passio* of Pavia. We know nothing of the conditions regarding this donation. Did the actual name of the messuage lead the monks to acquire it, and the donor to present it to them? Or, conversely, was it the donation that caused the monks of Cluny to be interested in Saint Guinefort?

Another document from Cluny, the *Chronicum cluniacense*, adds relevance to these two questions. It was a compilation from the end of the fifteenth century, which reproduced a number of earlier documents, and in particular the act of dedication of the third Abbacy of Cluny, in 1131.[10] This act lists the Abbey church's twenty-six altars amongst which, in the seventeenth position, we find the altars of Saint Leger and Saint Guinefort (*S.S. Leodegarii et Guineforti*). I can offer no explanation for this, but merely note that there is an association in the Cluny liturgy, between these two martyred saints. Saint Leger, Bishop of Autun, was martyred around 677–80. His feast day is 2 October.[11]

It seems quite probable that the cult of Saint Guinefort (*Guinifortus, Guinefortus, Guinefortis*) began to be diffused to the West of the Alps from the end of the eleventh century (Allevard, 1082) and during the twelfth century (Cluny, 1131), issuing from Pavia (which the *Passio* designates as the cult centre), and with the help of the monks of Cluny.

There is nothing particularly surprising about the exceptional prestige enjoyed by Pavia during this period, for around 1000 Pavia was the most important city in North Italy. Not only was it a monarchical centre, but it also had workshops for the minting of coins, a busy merchant class enjoying exorbitant privileges, and it was situated on the crossroads of various commercial routes. Pavia traded with the South of the peninsula, with Venice and the Adriatic, and with the countries over the Alps. In the first half of the eleventh century, Pavia's preeminence was shaken by the decline of the monarchy in Lombardy and by the rise of the new commercial centres, such as Milan, Cremona, Piacenza. But there was still very intense trading, particularly between Pavia and the South-East of Gaul, by way of Susa, Mont-Cénis, and the valleys of the Arc and the Isère.[12]

Now, religious, or, more properly, monastic relations were at least as old and intense as trading ones. From 999, Cluny reckoned Pavia as one of its most ancient priories.[13] The road between the two was dotted with still more priories and, from the eleventh century, with place names and cult sites dedicated to Saint Guinefort. Did the monks of Cluny take the name of Saint Guinefort to the peasants of the Dombes?

This question may seem, *a priori*, a surprising one. For the world of traditional monasticism and of the liturgical fasts that take place in the precinct of the cloisters, and that of the peasants, are normally, and quite rightly, considered to be quite alien to each other. It would be wrong, however, to see them as utterly distinct, for the monastery lived off the peasants' labour, and therefore necessarily entered into contact with them. The famous work *De miraculis* is proof enough of the openness of the monastic milieu to folk culture, and its author, Peter the Venerable, Abbot of Cluny between 1122 and 1156, collected a large number of narratives in order to assimilate them into the learned culture.[14]

A document from Cluny that was less well known in the twelfth century, and to which I have already alluded, is even more pertinent here. It is a narrative of the *circumvectio* of the relics of Saint Taurinus, borne in a procession, in 1158, by the monks of the Cluniac priory of Gigny (Jura). This narrative, which directly concerns the Dombes, makes it easier to understand how cultural and religious relations between monks and peasants might have been established, and how the latter might have heard tell, from the lips of the former, of Saint Guinefort.

Their priory having been destroyed by lightning, the monks of Gigny carried the relics of Saint Taurinus in procession. They hoped, by singing

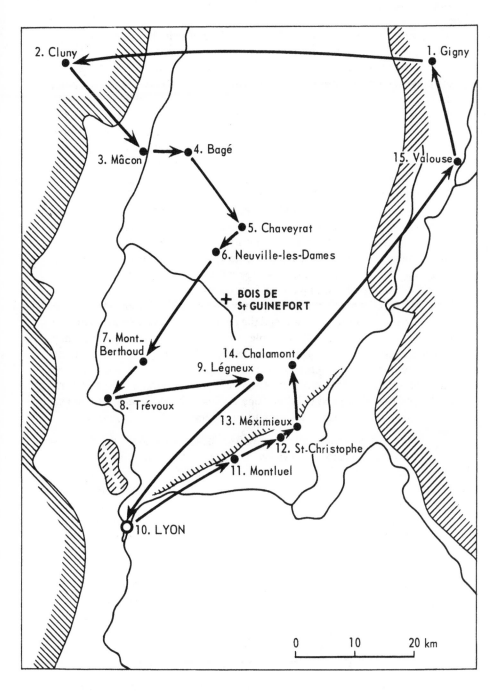

Map 2 *Circumvectio* of the relics of Saint Taurinus by the monks of Gigny, 1158
(*Acta sanctorum*, August II, 650–6) (Graphics Laboratory of the E.H.E.S.S.)

the saint's praises, and thanks to the miracles which the shrine might occasion, to obtain the offerings necessary for the reconstruction of their church. Such processions were common enough in the Middle Ages.[15] In the present case, the monks made first for the West, to the Abbey of Cluny, upon which they were dependent (see Map 2). Their periplus then took them South, towards the Dombes. Between Neuville-les-Dames and the Cluniac priory of Mont-Berthoud, where they halted, they must have passed very close to the spot where, less than a century later, Stephen of Bourbon went to suppress the cult of Saint Guinefort. Upon arriving at Lyons, they set out again towards the North-East, following the Eastern limit of the plateau of the Dombes, and then made their way back to Gigny. They made fifteen marches in all, covering an average of fifteen kilometres between halts (ranging, in fact, from three to thirty kilometres). At each halt, the monks lauded the saint's merits before the assembled populace, and numerous miracles occurred. Almost all of these involved healing, generally of women. Of the thirty-three miracles that are described in any detail (it also mentions, in passing, innumerable others), women were the beneficiaries of some sixteen, men of only eleven, and children of three. The three remaining miracles concerned the elements, or else animals. Thus, at Bâgé, the relics quieted a storm, while at Légneux a terrifying storm sprang up when its inhabitants refused to receive the relics, and at Chalamont some flies were miraculously prevented from polluting the shrine. Of the three miracles that benefited children, two were unexceptional, involving the healing of two paralysed children (one at Bâgé, the other at Chalamont). The third, at Lyons, takes us back to the theme of the *exemplum*:

> There was a man called Heldinus, whose only son, whilst still in his cradle, was struck down by so grave an illness that for five whole days he could neither sleep nor suck at his mother's breast. The heat of life had gone out of the child's limbs and only the faintest breath could be heard. The child's parents had, so to speak, exposed him (*eum tamquam exposuerant*). But his nurse, whose faith and devotion were ardent, decided to take the child to Saint Taurinus, and then to bring him back. Better still, she was moved to act and took the child to the saint, even though he was already thought to be dead. No sooner had the child been presented than he opened his eyes. Then he yawned and fell into a deep sleep. Then he howled, started to improve, and greedily emptied his mother's breast. So great a miracle was it that his father and mother, along with numerous neighbours, hastened to give praise to the greatness of God and to glorify the works of Saint Taurinus.

Many of these themes are reminiscent of Stephen of Bourbon's *exemplum*, namely the nurse and the suckling, the separation of the child from his parents, the theme of infanticide, the hopes of being saved *in extremis*. Although a hundred years separates them, these two testimonies show how enduring is the sentiment of anxiety that a sick child inspires (although his parents showed no hesitation, in this case, in exposing him), as also the expectation of a miraculous cure.

This narrative of a *circumvectio* also enables us to appreciate just how deeply Christianity, from the middle of the twelfth century, was rooted in the countryside, even if we take into account the tendency of monks to exaggerate the successes of their saint, and the ambiguity of certain attitudes. Thus the peasants of Bâgé undoubtedly attributed the cure of a paralysed person as much to the old oak under which the shrine was placed as to the saint's relics. But, having heard the monks sing the praises of Saint Taurinus, they would not be likely to have forgotten his name too quickly. And might not the monks have talked of yet other saints upon such occasions? Can we presume that there were other forms of contact between the peasants and the Cluniac monks? The 1158 *circumvectio* does at least show how the Cluniacs might, in the twelfth century, have made the name of Saint Guinefort known to the peasants of the Dombes.

Local testimonies of a much more recent date would seem to suggest that the various references to Saint Guinefort that we have traced all derive, in some form or other, from Cluny. Four other cult sites are recorded between the Saône and the Ain in the seventeenth and nineteenth centuries. Every one of them is in fact on the road that we have already followed from Pavia to Cluny, passing by way of Allevard and the banks of the Chalaronne, across the Dombes and through Tournus.

At the beginning of the eighteenth century, and in the vicinity of Tournus, upon the 'mountain of Saint Guillaume', the hermitage of Saint Guinefort (or Guy le Fort, or Guille le Fort) was founded, and young people came to consult the hermit about their marriage prospects.[16] In spite of the different forms that the name assumes, one can clearly recognise Saint Guinefort here. But it is worth noting how readily this name has become confused with that of other saints, in this case that of Saint Guy, a martyr, whose feast day was 15 June. Mere phonetic slips may account for such confusions, but I doubt if this explanation would hold good in every case, and a more systematic comparison of the saints involved, taking into consideration their names, status, functions, and feast days, should enable us to understand better how and why these slips occur.

In the last century, at Marlieux (Ain), a dozen kilometres to the East of Châtillon-sur-Chalaronne, women who wanted to have a child had to shake certain cherry trees whilst invoking 'Saint Guinefort'.[17]

Saint Guinefort was also known at Crêches (Saône-et-Loire, an *arrondissement* in Mâcon) at the end of the nineteenth century.[18] Finally, at Béreins, on the left bank of the Saône, some kilometres to the South-West of

Châtillon-sur-Chalaronne, the chapel (which has now been turned into a barn) of a manor (the only remains of which are some ruins built into the walls of a modern farm) was formerly dedicated to Saint Guinefort. The cult was still active at the time of the Revolution, and mothers in the nineteenth century still took their children there.[19]

It is thus possible to identify a series of sites dedicated to the cult of Saint Guinefort, extending from the right bank of the Saône (Cluny, Tournus, Crêches) to the Ain and the Isère (Allevard), and at the centre of which we find, on the banks of the Chalaronne, the one described in Stephen of Bourbon's *exemplum*. These testimonies are so numerous, and the saint's name is in each case so similar, that this series would seem to have a real unity. This impression is confirmed by the probable influence, at the start, of Cluny. But differences over devotional form were already emerging. At Cluny, the cult was integrated into the monastic liturgy, whereas in the Dombes, in the thirteenth as in the nineteenth century, it was invariably a folk cult. But nowhere else but in Stephen of Bourbon's *exemplum* is Saint Guinefort presented in the guise of a dog, and nowhere else but in Pavia does Saint Guinefort seem to have had a particular feast day, namely 22 August.

The saint's feast day is, in other places, the surest means we have of discovering how the cult of Saint Guinefort at Pavia came to be diffused. This is the case with the town of Puy, in the seventeenth century.

The church of Saint Michael, built in the tenth century, crowns the summit of the famous Aiguille ('Needle'), but in those days, at the foot and half way up, there were two chapels dedicated to two other archangels, Saint Raphael and Saint Gabriel. Now, according to the testimony of the Jesuit Odon of Gissey, on 22 August 1625 – the feast day of Saint Guinefort of Pavia – the Bishop of Puy

> consecrated the altar of the oratory of Saint Guinefort, which was perched on the rock of Saint Michael, after having enclosed in it the relics of Saint James the Apostle and of Saint Consortia. Just as before, on 28 April in the same year, he had consecrated the altar of the chapel of Saint Raphael, which was near to Saint Guinefort, having there enshrined some fragments of the bones of Saint John the Baptist, Saint Consortia and of certain holy martyrs. Posterity will be ever indebted to Canon André, who spared no expense in the embellishment of the church of Saint Michael and of the chapel of Saint Gabriel, let alone the costs he incurred in raising the altars and oratories of the Saints Raphael and Guinefort, in order to foster the ancient devotion there is upon this devout rock of the Aiguille.

The author then takes this opportunity to recall the legend of Saint Guinefort, of his brother 'Guinebolde', and of their sisters 'Pusilana' and 'Janila'.[20] There can be no doubt whatsover that this is the same saint as features at Pavia. This evidence as to the cult's diffusion is all the more remarkable for its being prior to the finding and translation of the body to the Monasterio Nuovo in 1650. It was only at this date that the dispersal of the relics began. The Bishop of Puy could therefore not have possessed any of them in 1625, and in consecrating the altar of the chapel of Saint Guinefort, on his feast day, he had to place relics of other saints beneath the altar stone.

There was certainly nothing arbitrary in the association between all these. For, between the church of Saint Michael, at the summit, and the chapel of Saint Gabriel, at the foot of the Aiguille, there was added, thanks to the generosity of a canon, a new chapel. It stood half way up, and was dedicated to the third Archangel, Saint Raphael. All three have feast days on 29 September. The relative heights of the different chapels represented a kind of inscription, in the rock itself, of gradations in the celestial hierarchy, from Gabriel, the angel of the Annunciation, and Raphael, healer and patron of travellers, to Michael, who subdued the dragon and guided the souls of the dead. Saint Guinefort, a healer like Raphael, who came to the aid of the dying, and who was associated with Saint Michael through the miracle at Péra, would have had no trouble in finding a place in this triad.

The choice of relics cannot have been fortuitous either. Saint James of Compostella, long venerated at Puy, a starting point for one of his pilgrimage routes, was himself a psychopomp. It was the miraculous birth of Saint John the Baptist that the archangel Gabriel had announced to Elizabeth and Zacharias. The presence of relics of Saint Consortia, a virgin, who was much venerated at Cluny, is less easy to explain. But it is worth noting that her feast day is 22 June, at the beginning of the summer, just like those of all the other saints who have been mentioned. Thus, Saint John the Baptist's feast day is 24 June, Saint James the Elder's (otherwise known as the Apostle) is 25 July, Saint Guinefort's 22 August, and the three archangels' 29 September. This dense liturgical grouping would seem to place even more emphasis on the relation between Saint Guinefort and the hot season.

We know, moreover, how important the cult of the three archangels, and of Saint Michael in particular, was to Cluny and to its dependents. Since the cults of Saint Consortia and Saint Guinefort were also, as we have seen, linked to this order,[21] might they not be the delayed effect of a Cluniac tradition?

At Puy, the chapel of Saint Guinefort has now disappeared. But at Le Velay, some forty kilometres from Puy, Saint Guinefort was still venerated in the nineteenth century, although in a quite different fashion. At the edge of a copse overlooking the river there stood a cross of white wood, and every Sunday, the peasants would take their sick babies to this place. Taking off the cloth in which the child was wrapped, and throwing it over the arms of the cross, they would say in a loud voice:

> Saint Guinafort, pour la vie, pour la mort.

If the linen still hung from the cross, the child would be saved. But if it fell to the earth, the child was 'doomed to a certain and imminent death'.[22]

During this same period, in the vicinity of Saint-Pardoux-Corbier (Corrèze), there was a fountain dedicated to the saint (*Fount Sent-Guinhe-Loufort*), with a cross that sickly (F.: *chétif*; O.F.: *chestis*) visitors had to walk round twice. The formula was identical:

> Saint Guinhe-lou-fort
> La vita ou la mort.[23]

The convergence of these folk cults raises various problems. What, for instance, was their relation to the popular forms in use at the cult in Pavia, and why, in particular, was there an identical formula for invoking the saint, i.e., 'for life or for death'? There is also the problem of the relation between the folk cult on the banks of the Lignon and the official cult at Puy. Had this latter become ruralised and folklorised?

At Saint-Junien (in Upper Vienne), the cemetery chapel, which dates from the thirteenth century, has a crypt which is said to be dedicated to Saint Guinefort, and which the bishop ordered to be closed in 1741. Since then, pilgrims have placed offerings in a small opening in the wall, which were dedicated to the sick, and to children. Excavations, conducted between 1966 and 1970, have uncovered numerous coins, of low denomination, and dating from the fifteenth to the twentieth century, as well as linen, shoes, pins and buttons.[24]

The above evidence from the Auvergne and from Limoges is the southernmost that I have encountered. Further to the North, Berry contains another group of cult sites, some of which are very old.

Between 1073 and 1078, a charter of donation intended for the collegiate church of Saint Ursinus at Bourges invokes 'the merits of the saints who rest [in this church]: Saint Ursinus first Archbishop of Bourges, Saint Sulpicius Severus, Saint Arcadius, Saint Justus, Saint Guinefort (Sanctus Guinefortis), Saint Rudolph'. The charter was drawn up on the occasion of a young knight taking the habit. The lord of Bourbon, Archambaud II the Younger (*c.* 1034–*c.* 1078) sanctioned the donation.[25]

The charter does not merely mention the saint, it also refers to the presence of the body of Saint Guinefort at Bourges, from the end of the eleventh century. Various proceedings of translation imply that the body was still present as late as 1648, 1668 and 1735.[26] In 1724, two monks of the congregation of Saint Maurus saw the body of Saint Guinefort when they visited Saint Ursinus at Bourges:

> Monsieur Alabat, who is its prior, showed me all the features of interest: the bodies of Saint Ursinus and of Saint Sulpicius Severus, which are kept behind the great altar, that of the abbot Saint Guinefort, who was formerly in a hollow altar and who has been transferred, a fine bust of the head of Saint Ursinus, and a relic of Saint Symphorian.[27]

It seems hard to reconcile this evidence with what we already know of the presence of Saint Guinefort's body at Pavia. Was the saint's body 'invented' in two different places? Or are two different saints involved? We must look into the matter more closely.

As the 1724 document shows, Saint Guinefort passed muster at Bourges as an 'abbot' rather than as a 'missionary and martyr', as at Pavia. Some nineteenth-century sources specify that he was a former abbot of the monastery of Saint Satur, near Sancerre, where he had a feast day on 27 February. There was even a parish named after 'Saint Généfort',[28] which was dependent upon this community. But no abbot of this name appears in the list that was maintained, uninterruptedly, from the restoration of the Abbey in 1034 by the Countess Ermengarde, the Archbishop of Bourges, and Archambaud II of Bourbon.[29] Another tradition, admittedly, considers Saint Guinefort to be a former abbot of Saint Symphorian at Bourges, a monastery which was responsible for the foundation of the collegiate church of Saint Ursinus.[30] Now, Saint Symphorian's feast day is 22 August, i.e., the day upon which Saint Guinefort was honoured at Pavia. Is this simply a coincidence, or can we posit a lasting relation between Pavia and Bourges, such that the cult, which was first celebrated in August, was then transferred (as was often the case) to the opposite end of the calendar, to February? Such duplication of feast days would explain why Saint Guinefort, who is honoured in Berry on 25, 26, and 27 February, when a specific feast day is mentioned, is also invoked at the collegiate church of Saint Martin at Levroux (in Indre) for the cure of 'Saint Sylvanus's fire', which is associated with the summer (Saint Sylvanus's feast day is 22 September).

However difficult it is to substantiate such an account of the cult's origin, one can still hazard a guess as to how, in the eleventh and twelfth centuries, the local cult developed, and how it was supported by the ecclesiastical foundations of Berry and by the seigneurial family of the Bourbons, which was then expanding rapidly.[31] This is borne out by the sheer number of places in Berry at which the saint was invoked in recent times. These were, for the most part, sites at which the folk cult was practised:

> Those poor invalids who can neither live nor die, and whom evil
> holds too fast, address Saint Guinefort (25 February) and cry:
> Grand saint Genefort!
> A la vie ou à la mort![32]

Sometimes his cult was associated with a chapel (at the manor of Chapelle-
d'Angillon, at Valigny-le-Monial, at Sancoins) or with a chapel of ease (at
Méry-ès-Bois). Saint Guinefort was also the patron of the church at
Tortezais, and the one at Verneuil-sur-Igneraie even now has an old statue
of Saint Guinefort.[33] Yet further proof of the cult's vitality lies in its having
spread from Berry in the direction of the Paris Basin.

According to Abbé Lebeuf, Saint Guinefort was honoured in the Ile-de-
France, on 26 August, in the parish church of Piscop, close to Pontoise. The
famous eighteenth-century scholar adds:

> I believe that the cult was brought to this place by a Scottish lord.
> His legend, which has it that he was born in Scotland, that he went
> into France with Gunibolde, his brother, and with two of his sisters,
> and thence into Italy, where Gunibolde was martyred at Cumes
> [sic] and Gunifort at Milan, has been judged to be so erroneous by
> the Bollandists, to whom I sent it, that they have not deigned to
> mention it.[34]

We know, however, that the *Acta sanctorum* did finally give a place to Saint
Guinefort! But Abbé Lebeuf seems to have had access to a text different
from the one which was published, for the saint was held by him to have
come from Scotland (although the scholar may well have mistranslated the
name *Scotia*, i.e., Ireland), to have disembarked in France (whereas, in the
Passio, Germany alone was mentioned), and to have had a feast day on 26
rather than 22 August. The main thing, however, is that he does indeed talk
of the same saint as features at Pavia, and that the discrepancy regarding
dates is minimal. He also offers an explanation for the cult's presence at
Piscop, namely that the local lords, the Braques, who were in alliance with
the Stuarts, must have introduced it in the sixteenth century. I accept the
hypothesis that the cult was in fact diffused, but refuse to allow that one may
account for the saint's being honoured at Piscop in terms of events on the
other side of the Channel. In fact, on 24 April 1684, the curé at Piscop
solemnly accepted Saint Guinefort's relics, through the mediation of a
Trinitarian monk, who had been granted the right to hold them by the
Archbishop of Bourges.[35] The cult at Bourges, like the one at Pavia, was
therefore diffused, possibly in similar circumstances, upon the occasion of
translations of relics. The last of these occurred in 1668. Yet a diffusion of
this sort could not help but have involved some adaptation to local
conditions. Thus, at Piscop, Saint Guinefort's feast day was 27 February,

as at Bourges, and he is clearly not the abbot of Saint-Satur, but the martyr of Pavia. This is why the Italian saint must presumably have preceded the saint from Berry, and why the reputation of the former justified the acquisition of the latter's relics, even though the feast day was still at the end of August.

Does the saint from Berry also feature at Sens? This would seem not to be the case, for at Sens Saint Guinefort is called a 'confessor'. He is flanked by a brother, Saint Fort, 'bishop and confessor' (whose feast day, according to the *French Martyrology*, was 16 May), and by a sister, Saint Avelina, a virgin. Unknown anywhere else, the latter is supposed to have been the first abbess of a Benedictine monastery whose sanctuary later became the parish church of Saint-Maurice-de-Sens. It was in this church, in 1241, that Archbishop Gauthier Cornut exhumed the bodies of the three saints and on 26 February 1445, Archbishop Louis of Melun had them displayed in a worthier place, where they might 'be conspicuous for the numerous miracles they occasioned'. This date was not fortuitous, for the *Martyrology of Sénon* (seventeenth century) in fact informs us that the three saints' feast days were all, locally, 26 February.[36] Now, this date is also that of the feast of Saint Guinefort in Berry. This would seem to suggest that the cult had been transmitted from Bourges to Sens, allowing nevertheless for a perceptible modification of some of the saint's other features.

The reputations of Saint Fort, Saint Guinefort and Saint Avelina went far beyond the limited circle of the clergy of Sens. In the nineteenth century, local legends told of two holy brothers who were travellers and who, while passing through Sens, recognised their sister in an inn. Another tradition actually has it that they were natives of Sens.[37] But the success enjoyed by Saint Fort, well known elsewhere in France and in Bordeaux in particular, undoubtedly eclipsed that of his brother and sister. It was he who was most commonly invoked at Saint Maurice-de-Sens for the cure of children with rickets, and in the surounding area, he was the only one to be invoked at Malicorne (in association with Saint Blaise, a fellow patron of the church, whose feast day was 3 February), and at the 'fountain of Saint-Fort', whose waters were thought to cure the sick.[38]

There is another series of cult sites to the North-West of the Paris Basin, stretching from Picardy to Normandy. Thus, in 1660, Dom Claude Bruslé, 'monk, priest, and sacristan', of the Cluniac priory at Montdidier, near Amiens, drew up an *Inventory of Holy Relics* preserved in his church. His fairly systematic inspection of the sanctuary led to the discovery, behind a cupboard, of a shrine in the form of an arm of a cross, which was eaten away by damp but contained some small fragments of bone. The attached schedules made it possible to identify them as follows: 'Some of the bones of Saint Lugle and Saint Luglienne', 'Of Saint Stephen, first martyr', 'Of Saint

Guinefort, also a martyr and bishop', 'Of S. Quentin, martyr', and 'Of Saints Julian and Agapitus, martyrs'.[39]

Although a martyr, and revered by the Cluniacs, this Saint Guinefort is not the one from Pavia. For he bears, and for the first time, the title of bishop (even at Sens he was simply a 'confessor', whilst Saint Fort was the sole person to bear the former title). This title in fact identifies him with another saint, honoured locally from the fifteenth century onwards, Saint Millefort. These two saints have identical healing powers and very similar legends and names, the latter being commonly confused with at least two other saints, Saint Dignefort and Saint Wilgeforte.

According to a nineteenth-century oral tradition, Saint Millefort was a Scottish bishop who, fleeing from the persecution unleashed by a prince in his own country, took refuge in the North-West of France. But at La Bouvaque, near to Abbeville, some serfs in Scottish pay beheaded him. According to another version, he succeeded in hiding himself in the area of La Bouvaque, and in hiring out his services to a farmer. The farmer's wife, guessing him to be a priest, confessed to him. Becoming jealous, the farmer beheaded him and buried his body at the place where he had been murdered. Miracles then took place, and the farmer built a chapel there. A third version has it that the chapel was constructed in order to shelter the holy martyr's head. A fourth version, on the other hand, has it that the bishop came from Scotland in the seventh century, and out of humility entered the service of a colonist from Ponthieu. Sometimes he left his plough to its own devices, whereupon it would follow the furrow as if guided by an invisible hand, whilst the saint kneeled down to pray. But so perfect was his work that the other labourers became jealous and cut off his head with a ploughshare. The saint put back his head upon his shoulders, finished his work, brought back his plough and let his head fall at the feet of the terrified colonist. He buried him with full honours and punished those guilty of the misdeed.[40]

There is evidence of the cult of Saint Millefort at La Bouvaque from 1419, in which year the Mayor of Abbeville had the chapel rebuilt. It was much visited in the eighteenth century, and on 3 November in particular, that being the saint's feast day. Great numbers of nurses took their sick children to this chapel and had them sit three times upon a particular stone, entirely naked, so that they might be cured.

His cult also featured in several other places in this area. At La Neuville-sous-Corbie, Saint Millefort was the patron saint of a lazar-house. His statue was subsequently taken to the parish church, where it is to this day. The saint is dressed as a bishop, carries a martyr's palm, and has in his keeping two children, which a man and a woman are holding out to him. His feast day was on 6 September, or on the second Sunday in September.

Near Camps, in Amiénois, a hermit in the nineteenth century renovated a chapel that had been wrecked at the time of the Revolution, and established the cult of Saint Millefort there, with the aim of diverting the pilgrims from La Bouvaque. On the fifth Sunday after Easter there was a procession in honour of the 'protector of children', and that same day, in a chapel built in 1850 at Saint-Aubin-Rivière by the parents of a child cured at La Bouvaque, a mass was celebrated.

This same cult also occurs in Normandy, for at Blangy (in Seine-Maritime) a chapel was dedicated to Saint Millefort. Tradition has it that he was martyred there. A pilgrimage for children stricken with 'listlessness' took place there every Shrove Tuesday. At Appeville (Eure) mothers would call upon Saint Millefort as recently as 1948, and would then scratch the stone of the pedestal of a statue, collecting the calcareous dust and mixing it with the milk in the infant's bottle, so as to fortify it.[41]

Saint Millefort was thus, like Saint Guinefort, a 'protector of childhood', and the confusion between the two saints is undoubtedly largely attributable to their having this function in common. At Golleville (Manche), on the main altar of the church, there is a statue of a bishop holding a martyr's palm, who, the inscription at the base would have us believe, is 'Saint Genefort'.[42]

Saint Guinefort has also been confused with Saint Dignefort, Bishop of Meaux and martyr, and for much the same reasons. From the second half of the fifteenth century, the Carmelites at Rouen and the members of Charité-Notre-Dame dedicated a cult to him. Because of the circumstances of his martyrdom, Saint Dignefort was often represented with his stomach open, and holding his intestines in his own two hands, and this is why, at Saussay-en-Caux, on 11 May (his feast day), he was invoked against the colic. But Saint Dignefort was, above all else, a protector of children. In the nineteenth century, at Gruchet-la-Valasse, he was invoked on behalf of children who were slow in learning to walk, and on 1 July, which was the day of the pilgrimage, mothers would strive to cross the procession between the cross and the banner, and would take their child several times round the church. They counted on curing their child in this fashion.[43]

These scattered references to Saint Dignefort help to explain why he has sometimes been confused with Saint Guinefort. A hesitation of this sort is, for instance, perceptible in Gonfreville-l'Orcher, in the eighteenth and nineteenth centuries, regarding the patron of the priory of Saint Dignefort, sometimes called Saint Guinefort.[44]

There have been similar confusions, in this same region, between Saint Guinefort and Saint Wilgeforte, or Guilleforte (in Latin, *Wilfortis* or *Wilgefortis*), virgin and martyr, whose feast day usually fell on 20 July. The legend has it that this daughter of a Portuguese king refused, because of her attachment to her faith and to her virginity consecrated to God, to marry the pagan king of Sicily. Hence the interpretation which is sometimes given of her name, 'steadfast virgin' (*vierge forte*), and her iconographic representation as a woman with a beard. We have evidence of this cult from the eleventh century onwards, in Flanders (under the name of Saint Kümmernis), in Holland (Saint Ontcommer), in England (Saint Uncumber). It spread from Flanders in the direction of Normandy. The same saint is also venerated in Aquitaine under the name of Saint Livrade (*Liberata*). The usual date of the feast day, 20 July, is observed in Normandy at Montpinçon (in the *canton* of Saint-Pierre-sur-Dives), and at Fauville (in the Yvetot *arrondissement*). At Daubeuf-Serville and at Vittefleur, the pilgrims gathered on 14 September instead. She was particularly concerned with retarded children, and with stomach upsets.[45]

At Arques, in 1607, a thirteenth-century chapel was rebuilt in honour of Saint Wilgeforte. However, in 1842, 'people went on pilgrimages there for those illnesses in which there was little hope of cure. They would leave a lighted candle, and make the following invocation in a loud voice: 'A Saint Guinefort, pour la vie ou pour la mort.' This meant that the sick person for whom one made the pilgrimage was bound either to recover or to die instantly, without further suffering.[46]

This formula is identical to the one we have already encountered in many other cult sites, Pavia included. Are we then to suppose that there is some connection between Saint Guinefort of Pavia, a native of Scotia, and Saint Millefort, *alias* Guinefort, a Scotsman from Normandy? This seems to me too fragile a hypothesis to be defended. But the Norman priest who, in 1896, had a relic of Saint Guinefort of Pavia bestowed upon his church was certainly in no doubt about this connection.

From Picardy and Normandy, where it is most strongly represented, the cult of Saint Millefort must have spread in the direction of the Ile de France. There is some sign of it in La Ferté-sous-Jouarre, to the North-East of Paris.[47] But, in this region too, Saint Millefort has been known to take the name of Saint Guinefort. Thus, at Bouillant parish church (Oise, in the *canton* of Crépy-en-Valois), there is a stone plinth bearing the inscription:

> S. Guinefort martyr
> Qui guérissés des
> Langueurs. prié
> Pour nous.
>
> (S. Guinefort, martyr
> Who curest
> lassitude, pray
> For us.)

The statue that this stone supported, and against which those with a fever would rub their linen, was that of a bishop (Illustration 5). He was

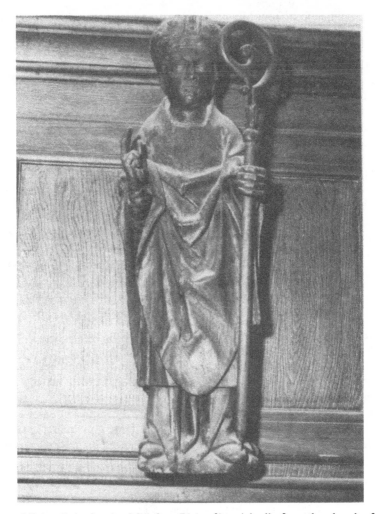

5 Statue of Saint Guinefort (or Millefort, Bishop?), originally from the church of Bouillant, Oise, but now in the care of the museum at Crépy-en-Valois

particularly invoked where it was a question of illnesses of the eye. Since this is a bishop and martyr, is he not in fact Saint Millefort?[48]

But we still have to explain why it is that, in the Ile-de-France and Normandy, the name of Saint Guinefort should have been given to Saint Millefort (and also, in the case of Normandy, to Saint Dignefort and to Saint Wilgeforte). The nature of the region may perhaps account for these confusions, for it is a contact zone between several cult areas. Saint Millefort's lies to the North-West (Picardy, Normandy), as does that of

Saint Dignefort (from Meaux to Normandy), and that of Saint Wilgeforte (Flanders, Picardy, Normandy). To the South-East we find the cult area of a Saint Guinefort, the one from Bourges, whose cult, as we have seen, extends in the direction of Sens, and even as far as Piscop itself. But can the other occasions upon which the name and cult of Saint Guinefort have been mentioned, in the Ile-de-France, be linked to this cult at Bourges?

Close to Dammartin-en-Goële, and not far from La Ferté-sous-Jouarre, there are references, in 1629 and 1637, to a farm, a chapel and an old lazar-house, which were all dedicated to Saint Guinefort.[49]

Likewise, in the eighteenth century, Abbé Lebeuf noted that the hamlet of Tigery, close to Corbeil, contained a chapel of Saint Guinefort or Genefort, situated on a farm belonging to the order of Saint John of Jerusalem:

> No offices are said there. But the farmer is obliged to have several masses said. Nor is the saint's feast day celebrated. But the inhabitants believe that when people did celebrate it, it was at the end of July . . . I saw on the altar a picture of two saints dressed in long robes. Behind this chapel, at a distance of eight to ten yards, there is a fountain in a little hollow. People make pilgrimages to it, and the water is said to be good for fever.[50]

Because people remember this feast day as having been at the end of July, Abbé Lebeuf, following Chastelain's *Martyrology*, takes 'Guinefort' to be a distortion of the name of Saint Cucuphas, a martyr, whose feast day in the diocese of Paris was 25 July. The latter, beheaded 'in the time of Diocletian', had had a cult long before in Barcelona, which was introduced to the Ile-de-France, in the ninth century, by the monks of Saint-Denis, at which point his name was sometimes changed into Quiquenfat or Guinefat. Hence the possibility of a confusion with Guinefort. Near Rueil, on the edge of the famous pool of Saint Cucuphas, there stood in the eighteenth century a chapel of Saint Quiqenfat,[51] the same saint who was honoured during the same period at Tigery, under the name of Saint Guinefort.

Is Chastelain's argument, as repeated by Lebeuf, at all convincing? I would hesitate to pass judgement one way or the other, and would simply note that a summer curative cult at Tigery, associated with a fountain, was placed, as elsewhere, under the patronage of Saint Guinefort.

There was also, finally, a group of cult sites in Brittany. I would emphasise the fact, first of all, that the name of Guinefort has there been given to a river, the Guinefort, which is a small tributary of the Rance.[52] Once again, then, we find this name associated with the theme of running water.

The saint himself was venerated in Brittany in three different places. At the beginning of the twentieth century, at Saint Broladre (the *canton* of Pleine-Fougères, Ille-et-Vilaine), there was a fountain and a ruined chapel dedicated to Saint Guinefort, and there one might see a wooden statue that innumerable coats of whitewash had rendered unrecognisable. When a child had long been ill, it was the custom to commend him to 'Saint Guinefort, qui donne la vie ou la mort.' The traditional rite went as follows. One placed the child's head in a hole in the wall, which was called a 'furnace'; if the child raised his head, it was a sign of life, but if he let it fall, the answer was 'death'. In the same canton, and as late as 1922, a chapel that had not been used since the Revolution was the object of a similar cult:

> Three stone statues have been preserved there, one dedicated to Saint Denis, the other to I know not whom, and the third to Saint Guinefort. Small pilgrimages are still made to this latter, and people pray for those who are dying, and who show too much resistance to it, that he should accord them 'life or death'.[53]

The presence of a statue of Saint Denis makes it tempting to compare this cult with that of Saint Cucuphas, as Chastelain's hypothesis suggests, but the argument is a fragile one.

Finally, the church of Saint Martin in Lamballe (Côtes-du-Nord) had, at the end of the nineteenth century, a statue of Saint Geufort or Guinfort or Généfort 'who gives life or death', particularly in relation to sick children:

> Saint Généfort has the face of a big baby; his right hand is extended, and in his left hand he bears a martyr's palm. The *ex-votos* are composed of rosaries, children's bonnets, figurines in white wax, crutches. That, a peasant who was in the church told me, is Saint Généor, who gives life or death. He is only to be invoked in extreme cases. He is kind enough to restore you to health immediately, or else to relieve you of your life immediately.

Another person gave the following account:

> When someone is dangerously ill, and is considered as good as lost, and when his state neither worsens nor improves, one invokes Saint Guinefort and one has a candle burned in his honour, and, if possible, in front of his picture, so that some change, be it for good or ill, might take place, which might be termed playing for double or quits. So it is that people always say:
> 'Saint Guinefort Pour la vie ou la mort'.[54]

The long trajectory in space and time that I have just described has produced forty references to Saint Guinefort or to his cult sites. But it has not proved simple. Scholars, very often clergymen themselves, have preferred to study the saints that the Chuch had already honoured the most. We hardly know which intellectual instruments to use in starting to enquire into an obscure saint of uncertain status (abbot, bishop, dog?). Some specific studies (by Maiocchi, Edouard, Corblet) have opened up a possible approach for us, and hagiographic lists (*Vie des saints et des bienheureux, Bibliotheca sanctorum*) provide valuable clues. But I have also had to ransack, and often fruitlessly, all the existing departmental topographic dictionaries and all the lists of place names drawn up by the administration of the Archives de France (typewritten volumes that are available in the reading room of the Archives Nationales in Paris). Given the means to hand, the enquiry has been as detailed and thorough as possible.

I have traced all existing references to 'Saint Guinefort'. But, truth to tell, this name appears in so many different forms that it is sometimes hard to know how to delimit the field of enquiry. In Latin, we have found Winifortus (a Germanic form which has been latinised, favoured by the Bollandists, but which we have never really encountered in texts), Guinifortus, Guinefortus, Gunifortus, Guinefortis. In Italian, we have found Guniforto, and, occasionally, Boniforto. In French, there is a very wide range of different names in use: Guinefort, Guignefort, Gunifort, Gueufort, Généfort, Guignafort, Guignefont, Guy-le-Fort, Guille-le-Fort. We have also had to take the names of other Saints, such as Millefort, Dignefort, Wilgeforte or Guilleforte, whenever they have been confused with Guinefort. One could also compare this latter name with the place name Guinefolle, which occurs in the West of France (Mayenne, Vienne, Sarthe, Loire-Atlantique). I ought finally to mention certain of the French forms of the name of Saint Cucuphas, i.e., Guinefat and Quinquenfat.

The forty references to Saint Guinefort which have been identified are scattered along a South-East/North-West diagonal, from North Italy to Picardy. These references belong, for the most part, to modern times (twenty-eight cases), but there are definite traces of a cult of Saint Guinefort from the eleventh century onwards (at Bourges, around 1075, and at Allevard, in 1082), in the twelfth century (at Cluny, in 1131), and in the thirteenth century (at Pavia, in 1236, at Sens, in 1241, in the Dombes, around 1250). The oldest evidence we have concerns the two zones situated to the South-East of our map, with a first series between the Po and the Saône, and a second centred on Bourges, and also on Sens. On the other hand, the most recent evidence (from the eighteenth to the twentieth century) concerns Normandy and Picardy (where the name of Saint Guinefort obscures the names of other saints), Brittany and the Ile-de-France.

It had seemed reasonable enough to begin by asking the questions that have been traditonally asked about the cult of saints: What is the origin of a particular cult? How was it diffused? The limitations of such an approach speak for themselves. But it was necessary to start there.

In order to establish a possible line of descent for the two main cult sites I employed the following criteria:

1. An explicit reference to a link between two cult sites, and particularly when it is attributable to the transport of relics from one place to the other, between Bourges and Piscop in the seventeenth century, for instance.
2. Geographical proximity, which enables one to define a series of cult sites as being grouped around a centre, Milan or Berry in particular.
3. Compulsory itineraries, marked out by so tight a chain of cult sites that it is a simple matter to guess the missing links, between Pavia, Allevard, the Dombes and Cluny, for instance.
4. Institutional connections, particularly in the case of a cult being subsumed by a particular religious order, as at Cluny. This criterion may reinforce the previous one, as in the case of relations between Pavia and Cluny.
5. Where relevant, the date of the saint's feast day. The feast day of 22 August enabled us to posit a connection between Pavia and Puy, and those of 25, 26 and 27 February enabled us to do the same for Bourges and Sens.
6. The status of saint. The name of 'martyr', given to the saint at Pavia, occurs again in the case of the greyhound in the Dombes who is cited in the *exemplum*, and, to my mind, implies that there is indeed, as criteria 3 and 4 suggest, a connection. The status of 'abbot' enables us to isolate the distinctive feature of the cult at Berry, whilst that of 'bishop' allows us to discern, beneath the name of Saint Guinefort, the cult of Saint Millefort.

In combining all these criteria, we arrive at a result very different from the one that we might have anticipated, for, rather than having identified the origin of a cult, the directions in which it was diffused, and the stages through which it passed, we have brought to light, behind the multiple forms of a single name, the cults of several saints. Table 4 presents their respective 'identity cards'.

Finally, we have found not just *one* Saint Guinefort, but at least two from the eleventh century onwards, not counting the more recent confusions that have arisen.

But Table 4 has its limitations, in that several references to the cult have not been linked with any certainty to one or other of the saints identified. This is the case with the three cult sites in Brittany, and that at Saint-Pardoux-Corbier, for neither the proximity of a particular group of cult sites nor the characteristics of the saint honoured locally (i.e., his status or his feast day) enable us to link them to other sites. These cases may not be subsumed within my typology, and it is quite comprehensible that this

Table 4 *The Saint Guineforts*

1. *Guinefort 'of Pavia'*
Name: Winifortus, Guinifortus, Gunifortus, Gunifortis, Guniforto, Boniforto, Guinefort
Status: martyr, missionary, greyhound?
Feast day: should the occasion arise, 22 August (26 August?, at Piscop)
Kin: a brother, Saint Guniboldus, martyr; two sisters: Saint Pusillana and Saint Favilla, martyrs
Localities: from the Po to the Saône and the Upper Loire
First definite reference: 1082

2. *Guinefort 'of Bourges'*
Name: Guinefort, Généfort
Status: abbé
Feast day: should the occasion arise, 25, 26, or 27 February
Kin: none
Localities: Berry, relics introduced at Piscop
First reference: 1073–8

The Sens variant (?)
Name: Guinefort
Status: confessor
Feast day: 26 February
Kin: a brother, Saint Fort, bishop and confessor, and a sister, Saint Avelina, abbess, virgin
Localities: Sens
First reference: 1241

3. *Millefort, alias Guinefort, and other instances of confusion*
Name: Guinefort, Généfort
Status: bishop and martyr
Feast day: never specified when the saint bears this name. Otherwise, 6 September (La Bouvaque), Sunday after Easter (Camps), Shrove Tuesday (Blangy)
Kin: none
Localities: Picardy, Normandy, Ile-de-France
First reference: by this name, 1660. Otherwise, 1419

Similar cases of confusion, in these same areas, in the eighteenth century
Dignefort (honoured on 11 May or 1 July)
Wilgeforte (honoured on 20 July)
Cucufat (honoured on 25 July)

should be so. The criteria employed in establishing this typology derive, for the most part, from the learned culture's hagiography. This means that those folk cult sites at which the saint is celebrated throughout the year, and not upon a particular feast day, and in which his official status is not specified, are *de facto* eliminated. The most distinctive features of the folk cult sites are therefore quite different, but, *irrespective of the saint's identity*, they are to be found as much in Berry as in Normandy. These are as follows:

1. The formula of invocation: 'A Saint Guinefort, pour la vie ou la mort'. I have found this at six different cult sites, at Pavia (Chi si vota a S. Boniforto, dopo tre giorni è vivo o morto'), on the banks of the Lignon (S. Guignafort, pour la vie, pour la mort'), at Saint-Pardoux-Corbier ('Saint Guinhe-Lou-Fort, La vita ou la mort'), in Berry ('Grand Saint Genefort, à la vie ou à la mort'), at Arques, in a place of pilgrimage dedicated originally to Saint Wilgeforte ('A Saint Guinefort, qui donne la vie ou la mort'), at Saint Broladre, Roz-sur-Couesnon and Lamballe ('A Saint Guinefort, qui donne la vie ou la mort'). This formula scarcely alters from place to place, no matter how large a distance is involved, and has been found even fairly recently. But, at a much earlier period, we also find a trace of it in Stephen of Bourbon's *exemplum*, which also describes a folk cult of Saint Guinefort. The formula itself is not quoted, but the final stage of the rite could not possibly signify anything else: 'if it came through without dying on the spot, or shortly afterwards, it had a very strong constitution'. The alternative is the same as is uttered elsewhere, in the saint's formula of invocation.

2. The saint tends to be invoked on behalf of two categories of patients: those who, on the point of death, neither die nor recover, and therefore one asks the saint to decide what their destiny is to be; and children, whose condition is sometimes a desperate one, but who often simply suffer from benign afflictions, e.g. 'lassitude' or 'fever', or who are just slow in learning how to walk ('knotted' children). It is true that the slightest disease could worsen rapidly and have fatal consequences for them.

3. Folk cult sites are almost invariably in the same sort of places. They are often country chapels, preferably isolated, and sometimes adjoining a hermitage (Tournus, in the seventeenth century), a malarial hospital (Tigery, in the eighteenth century), or a lazar-house (Dammartin). A statue, which is usually difficult to identify, is sometimes kept there (Saint Broladre). The rites which are enacted contravene ecclesiastical rules, although they are also to be found in the great sanctuaries of Christianity in the Middle Ages:[55] the faithful scrape the stone and gather up the dust from it, they place the sick child's head in a hole in the wall (the 'furnace') or, as in the *exemplum*, between the trees in the wood. The cult site often features a fountain or a river (in Stephen of Bourbon's *exemplum*, and also at Saint Broladre, Tigery, Saint-Pardoux-Corbier, on the banks of the Lignon; and, in Brittany, there is actually a river bearing the saint's name).

4. Whereas, in those cult sites that were most under the control of the clergy, the saint's feast day was on a particular day of the year (as at Pavia and Piscop), the folk cult was generally operative throughout the year, even when it was associated with a chapel. On the other hand,

where a cult had no clerical features whatsoever (no statue or chapel), and where the folk rites of contact or immersion were to the fore, as at Saint-Pardoux-Corbier, on the banks of the Lignon, at Marlieux or in Stephen of Bourbon's *exemplum*, no annual feast day was mentioned.

I shall now propose a new typology, one which takes account of the cult's forms and functions, which obviously transcends the distinction between the various saints, and which has the advantage of subsuming all the cult sites that have been identified. This time I shall distinguish between:

1. An official, clerical, and often even monastic form of the cult. It is linked to the altar of a church, it often entails the veneration of relics and the exaltation of a saint's statue upon the occasion of his annual feast day. At this level, the distinction between several Saint Guineforts can, and indeed ought to, be made. The oldest instances of the cult (at Pavia and Bourges) are usually of this order.
2. An intermediate form, controlled by a member of the clergy (a chaplain) or simply by a hermit, who would be attached to a country chapel. The latter sometimes contains a statue that tradition identifies as being that of Saint Guinefort, and which is the object of folk rites. An annual pilgrimage is sometimes held, on a fixed date. This form of the cult is heavily documented in the seventeenth and eighteenth centuries, and also in the last century.
3. A thoroughly folkloric form, which ruled out any clerical control but not therefore actual references to Christianity, since it was invariably a saint who was venerated (even if it was a dog), and since Christian symbols, the cross for instance, might well be present. Relics, chapels, statues and fixed feast days were excluded. Nature, whether wooded or aquatic, was the framework for the cult. Without the observations of folklorists in the nineteenth century, and in the first half of the twentieth century, we would not know of this cult, were it not for a single exception, namely Stephen of Bourbon's *exemplum* in the thirteenth century.

The reader will have noticed that the testimonies regarding these three cult forms are unevenly distributed over the different historical periods. In fact, the more official the cult is, the more ancient is the documentation respecting it; whereas the more folkloric it is, the more chance there is of its appearing in the most recent documents. Can one explain this distribution over time of the various cult forms in terms of a continuous and general process of folkorisation of the official cults of several saints, occurring in modern times and tending, moreover, to result in the gradual loss of their distinctive features? This may well be true of the area around Puy, and it is certainly the case with the area around Bourges. But more commonly it is changes in the rate of documentation which give rise to the illusion of a diachronic transformation of the cult. The folk cult described by Stephen of Bourbon is as old as many of the official cults, and if it is the result of a folklorisation of the Cluniac cult, this transformation occurred well before the modern period.

Two different forms may in fact coexist in the same place and in the same period, as is the case, in recent times, with Pavia.

One ought not, therefore, to draw too great a distinction between the forms, be they predominantly folkloric or predominantly official, of the cult, for there have been both diachronic and synchronic relations between the two. But, however much contact there may have been, one cannot help but acknowledge the existence of distinct and largely autonomous cultural networks, within which information is transmitted in a closed circuit. One of these networks was Cluniac. The network of folklore and of oral tradition undoubtedly functioned in a more restricted manner.

The notion of a network enables us to understand why Stephen of Bourbon should have been so astonished at hearing tell of Saint Guinefort, whose name was unknown to him. Yet he was born on the opposite bank of the Saône, which was close by, and he had, in the guise of inquisitor, patrolled the whole region. But he was a clergyman who had studied at Paris, and the folk culture was foreign to him. He was also a Dominican, a child of the town and of scholasticism, and he was not too familiar with Cluniac traditions, or with the old rural monasticism.

8

THE ETHNOGRAPHIC ENQUIRY IN THE DOMBES

Stephen of Bourbon had hoped, by repressing the cult of Saint Guinefort, dog and martyr, on the banks of the Chalaronne, to prevent the pilgrimage ever being revived. The dog's bones were burned, as was the wood, and the peasants were threatened with the confiscation of their goods if they relapsed. The cult would seem to have been definitively destroyed. Which is why this episode, culminating as it did in a total success for the church, became an *exemplum*. Other preachers might then use it as evidence for the fact that the faith, in its fight against superstition, would not be satisfied with half measures.

Yet this pilgrimage still seems to have been in existence in 1826. We learn this from another cleric, and, for all the centuries that had passed, his language was remarkably similar to that of Stephen of Bourbon.

In 1823, during the Restoration, and a year after the reinstatement of the diocese of Belley (which the Concordat of 1790 had suppressed), the new Bishop, Monsignor Devie, wishing to acquaint himself with his diocese, sent to each *commune*, and to each curé, a fairly detailed questionnaire concerning the material and spiritual circumstances of his parishioners. All the curés were requested to return the completed questionnaires. A subsequent enquiry, using the same questionnaires, took place in 1825. Questions covered the material state of the church and benefice, the liturgical observances and cult objects, the moral and educational level of the curé's assistants, the piety of the parishioners etc. The questionnaire was four pages long, and at the end there was a space left free so that the curé might add any further observations. The answers were then reclassified by *commune, arrondissement* and *canton*, and bound into two large volumes which may still be seen today at the Bishop's library at Belley (in the *département* of Ain).[1]

One of the questions was formulated as follows: 'What superstitions are current in the parish?' The answers are disappointingly brief, although this may have been due to lack of space. But the final heading, 'Observations', gave the priests an opportunity to say a good deal more about this subject. This heading gave them more room to describe the folk practices with which, in some cases, they were very familiar, having tried in vain to eradicate them. Whenever a curé used this heading it was almost invariably to speak of 'superstitions', for the ordinary headings normally sufficed to answer the questions. However, those answers and observations which had to do with the *communes* on the banks of the Chalaronne make no mention of a cult of Saint Guinefort, either as dog or as man. If we just had these two enquiries, we would doubtless suppose that Stephen of Bourbon's efforts had been entirely successful.

But, in the register of the 1823 enquiry, a letter is appended to the answer of the curé from Châtillon-sur-Chalaronne. It had been sent from Brou, on 17 September, 1826, by the curé of Châtillon, one Dufournet, to the Bishop of Belley. This letter alluded to another one, which I have failed to discover, and which a mendicant must have sent to the bishop. The bishop would seem to have informed the curé of the mendicant's actions, and to have asked for further information. The curé answered as follows:

[*Verso*] Monsignor,

Monsignor the Bishop of Belley,

residing at present at the Seminary of Brou

[*Recto*]   *Brou, 17 September, 1826*

Monsignor,

I am answering a letter that a mendicant, who has been resident for the last two or three years in a wood of M. Duchatelard's not far from Châtillon, has sent you, asking you if he might establish a kind of chapel there.

This man has taken up residence in M. Duchatelard's wood without his permission. What is more, fearing that he may set fire to his woods and noting with some anxiety the number of people that the mendicant has attracted, M. Duchatelard greatly desires that he should betake himself elsewhere, but has no wish to deal too severely with the wretch.

I think that this wretch only means to make a kind of living there, and to use the pretext of a religion he barely understands in order to obtain alms. He claims to have discovered a saint in this wood, and that he knows the site where he is buried. I very much doubt this, unless he means some stone statue or other. He has assembled some fragments of little wooden or stone statues, which he has placed in a little chapel, which he has decorated as best he can with foliage, and it is there that a fair number of people go in order to give him things.

People have long been visiting this wood in honour of Saint Guinefort. Mothers with ailing children come from far and near. Those with a fever come too, and tie or knot a little branch from a tree, and claim thus to knot the fever. This, Monsignor, is all I know of the subject.

I remain, your eminence, your very humble and obedient servant,

Dufornet, curé.

This letter was written quite independently of Stephen of Bourbon's evidence. Neither curé Dufournet, nor obviously the mendicant, nor even the Bishop of Belley knew of the *exemplum*. This only adds to the interest of the curé's letter. Does it prove that the cult which it describes is a continuation, in the very same place, of the one suppressed by the thirteenth-century inquisitor?

Curé Dufournet gives us a very exact description of the siting of Saint Guinefort's cult, namely, on M. Duchatelard's lands. The latter was Comte Jean-François Perret du Châtelard, owner of the manor at Clerdan, which he had just built. He died in 1843, and his nephew the Comte de la Rochette then succeeded him. According to the rector, the mendicant had established himself in the woods near to this manor, on the right bank of the Chalaronne. Two documents, older even than this letter, allow us to situate this wood yet more accurately.

A deed executed on 27 September 1632 mentions a plot of land 'bordered on the east by the mill-course of Crozo, and on the west by the hermitages upon which the chapels of Saint Guy le Fort used to stand'.[2]

The example of Tournus in the seventeenth century, which I mentioned above, confirms that this is undoubtedly Saint Guinefort's name here. Besides, the chapels named after him, and which would seem to have been, by 1632, no more than a memory, were to the West of a certain 'Crozo mill'. This mill is easily identified in the survey of 1811, which I consulted in Sandrans town hall and which, unlike the more recent survey, features the name 'Saint Guinefort's wood' among the plots of land bounded on the East by Crozo (or Crozat) mill, and on the South by the Chalaronne. This wood is situated at the furthest point West of the *commune* of Sandrans (Ain), as the 1857 map also shows (a small-scale version of which is reproduced here, Map 3). The wood is bounded on the South by the Chalaronne and on the East by the mill-course which allows 'Crosat pond' to flow into the river. It is in the only part of the *commune* of Sandrans which is to the North of the Chalaronne, at the point where this *commune* touches the neighbouring ones of Châtillon-sur-Chalaronne, Romans, La Chapelle-du-Châtelard, and even Saint-Georges-sur-Renom. This wood is about eight hundred metres, as the crow flies, from the manor of Clerdan, and it was undoubtedly there that the mendicant denounced by the rector Dufournet built his chapel. But is this wood also the one that Stephen of Bourbon described?

The following two arguments may be raised against this hypothesis. First, even supposing that one were to accept at face value the legend of the greyhound, such as Stephen of Bourbon heard and recounted it (and I shall come back to this point), it is still the case that no ruin remains. To which one could, admittedly, object that the presumed disappearance of the *castrum* occurred at least seven centuries ago. Secondly, if the mendicant, in 1823, claimed to know of a saint's burial place, and to dress up wooden and stone statuettes as saints, there was clearly no dog involved (a thing that the curé would undoubtedly have denounced in no uncertain terms to the bishop), but rather statues of saints in human form. One could nevertheless argue that the rector was not in touch with all that people said respecting this pilgrimage site, and that, being unaware of the existence of Stephen of Bourbon's *exemplum*, he had no motive for enquiring any further.

Those arguments which, on the other hand, would lead one to suppose that a cult had endured all that time on the same site, and in spite of Stephen of Bourbon's suppression of it, seem to me to be much more convincing. They are four in number.

The reader will recall how Stephen of Bourbon emphasised the part that the river Chalaronne played in the performance of the rite. The river would therefore have to be quite close to the trees where the first part of the rite took place. Now, 'Saint Guinefort's wood', which we have just located quite precisely, is but a few dozen metres from the Chalaronne. Furthermore, it is just where the Crosat mill-course flows into the river that it comes closest to the hills that fringe the river bed to the North-East. Downstream from the wood, on the other hand, it leaves this hillside and winds its way towards the South. An observer visiting the actual site cannot help but be struck not only by the proximity of the wood to the river, but also by their close interrelation. For the hill which the wood covers overlooks the river from a height of about ten metres, and slopes gently down towards it in a Southerly direction. It is a deciduous wood, with such dense and bushy undergrowth that it would be impenetrable, were it not for a path that allows one to enter and to climb the slope up to the top of the hill. The tree-trunks there are both more widely spaced and larger. The same path, on the way back, leads straight to the South, and in the direction of the river, at the very point where it runs closest to the foot of the hill (see Illustration 6).

The second argument rests on the sheer age of the cult of Saint Guinefort, which curé Dufournet, in 1826, had himself acknowledged ('People have long been visiting this wood in honour of Saint Guinefort. . .'), and which the deed executed in 1632 confirms. The letter refers, moreover, to a yet earlier period. It mentions 'chapels' which are supposed to have stood there 'formerly'. The fact that it refers to the possible existence of such chapels in the past seems to me to be more significant than their actual existence or otherwise. One may compare this formula with what is said, in the *exemplum*, of the *castrum* whose memory was kept alive by the peasants. In both documents, the memory of a building (whether 'true' or 'false', it matters little here) is an integral part of the folk representation of the site.

The parallel with the *exemplum* becomes all the more convincing when one recalls that 'the chapels of Saint Guy le Fort' must have stood, according to the deed of 1632, on the fallow land (*hermiture*) to the west of Crozo mill-course. We thus find, four centuries later, a word employed as

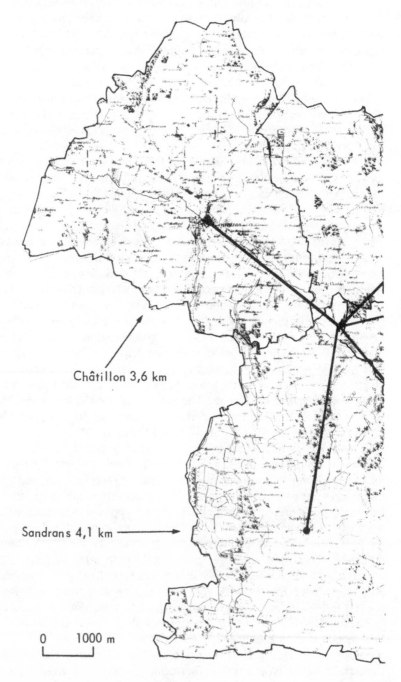

Châtillon 3,6 km

Sandrans 4,1 km

0   1000 m

Map 3 Situation of 'Saint Guinefort's wood' in the *commune* of Sandrans, Ain
(Graphics Laboratory of the E.H.E.S.S.)

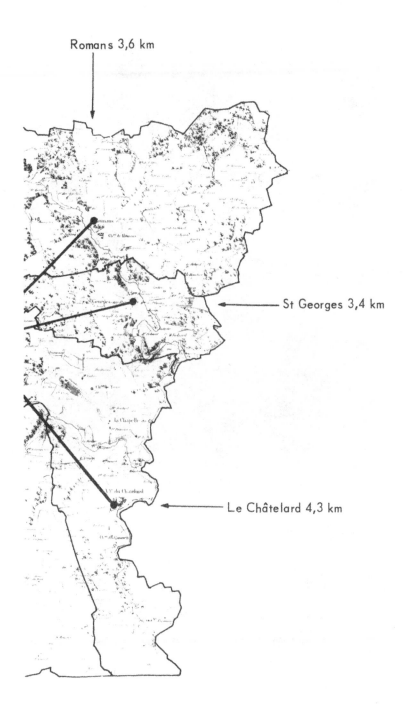

Romans 3,6 km

St Georges 3,4 km

Le Châtelard 4,3 km

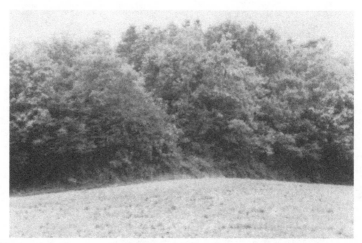

6 'Saint-Guinefort's wood' at Sandrans, Ain
  (a) The wood seen from the North. The path into it is clearly visible (August 1977)

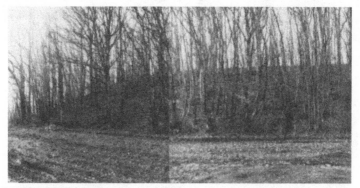

(b) The platform and the point of the spur, seen from the East (February 1978)

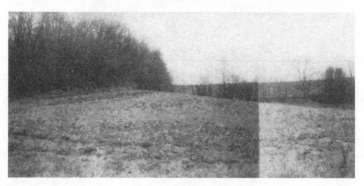

(c) The extreme tip of the spur, seen from the South-West (February 1978)

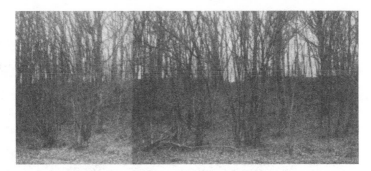

(d) The knoll and the ditch, seen from the North-East (February 1978)

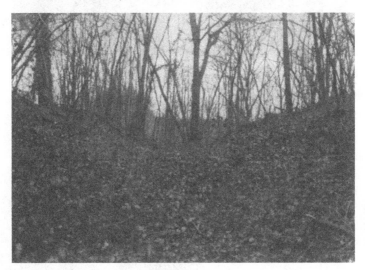

(e) Detail of the ditch (February 1978)

common noun (*hermitures*, i.e., fallow land) that Stephen of Bourbon had used as a place name (*silva de Rimite*). The fact that the land had for so long been designated by the same name suggests that the same site was involved in each case.

This hypothesis is further strengthened by a final argument, with regard to the distance separating this wood from the nearest localities. In a wooded terrain of this sort, the *communes* tend to be scattered around a more important site upon which, at a slight incline, a manor-house will usually stand. Now, the wood of Saint Guinefort is equidistant (*c.* four kilometres) from the five villages surrounding it, namely, Châtillon-sur-Chalaronne (3.6 km), Romans (3.6 km), Saint-Georges-sur-Renom (3.4 km), Le Châtelard (4.3 km) and Sandrans (4.1 km). This distance accords with

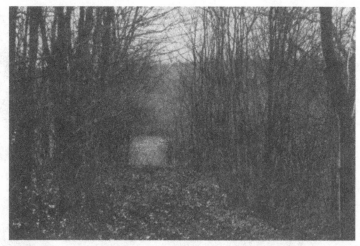

(f) Detail of the path, seen from inside the wood, and looking in the direction of the Chalaronne, towards the South

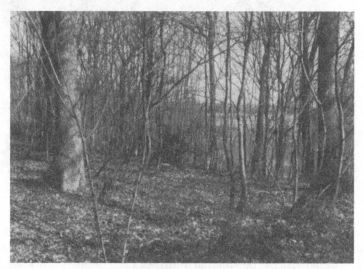

(g) The large trees at the top of the platform (January 1977)

Stephen of Bourbon's own assessment, that it was 'about a league (4.4 km)' between the *castrum* from which the witch came and the cult site beside the Chalaronne. Without arriving at a more precise identification of this *castrum*, it is worth noting that Sandrans, Châtillon, and Le Châtelard, because of the distance, because of their fortified appearance and (in the case of the last two) because of their names, would seem altogether to bear out my hypothesis.

The distance of the wood from these villages also helps to explain why it is that, with the exception of the deed of 1632, the documents are silent about it, from the middle of the thirteenth century to the beginning of the nineteenth century. This distance certainly did much to protect the cult site, isolated as it was in the woods and on the boundaries of five adjoining territories. For the representatives of the ecclesiastical powers to come to this place and give some concrete expression of their hostility towards this cult, they would have to have had a very specific and serious reason to travel there, let alone to take an interest in it. Stephen of Bourbon must have heard some remarkable things at confession to draw him so deep into the woods. On the other hand, if the Archbishop of Lyons, and then the Bishop of Belley (from the seventeenth century onwards), or their agents responsible for pastoral matters (whose reports have been preserved in large numbers from the fifteenth century onwards), also visited Sandrans, Châtillon-sur-Chalaronne, La Chapelle-du-Châtelard or Romans, they were only concerned with the clergy's education, with the revenues from the parish, or with the state of the buildings in the main church. Never once did they inspect all the parish lands, the chapels or the more distant cult sites. This is why none of the pastoral visits to one or to several of these parishes, in 1469, 1470, 1613, 1655, 1778 or 1784, mentions the cult of Saint Guinefort.[3] Even in 1823, when the Bishop of Belley asked about superstitions, the curé of Sandrans could only reply: 'The people around here are fairly superstitious, one in one way, and one in another.' And in 1825 he gave a similar answer regarding superstitions: 'They do not exist.' The curé at Châtillon-sur-Chalaronne was of the same opinion. When asked whether there were superstitions in his parish, he answered, in 1823, that there were 'None in particular, although various people believe in dreams and in other superstitions of that sort, as is the case everywhere.' And in 1825: 'They do not exist.' His letter of the following year was very different, but it was no longer a matter of answering a general enquiry. Following the mendicant's behaviour, the Bishop had asked the rector a very precise question about the cult of Saint Guinefort. Since he was not obliged to speak at once of all the superstitions with which he was familiar, he was free, in his letter to the Bishop, to enlarge upon one of them.

Thus, around 1250, and again in 1826, the documents' silence was broken, and in similar circumstances, namely at the initiative of ecclesiastical authorities outside the community and unfamilar with the folk culture.

In this respect, Curé Dufournet's letter is part of a long tradition of hostility between the clerical and folk cultures. But it also marks the end of it. When Saint Guinefort's cult resurfaces in the course of the nineteenth century, in written documents, the initiative still belongs to the learned culture, but the latter is no longer closely tied to the church and often actually turns its back on it.[4]

In 1877 Lecoy de la Marche published extracts from Stephen of Bourbon's treatise, among them the *exemplum* of Saint Guinefort. This narrative immediately aroused the interest of local folklorists: had they not found, if not the origins, at any rate very ancient evidence of practices that could still be witnessed? Their habitual approach was turned upside down, for, instead of beginning with a particular discovery, they had access to a guide, Stephen of Bourbon, and they wondered to what extent his observations and theirs might tally. They paid particular attention to the question of the saint's identity: was he a man or a dog? The ideological positions of these authors had not a little influence on the answers they gave to this question.

From 1879 onwards, Vayssière published the results of his researches. He had gone to 'Saint Guinefort's wood' and had gathered information about the cult:

> All those whom I approached told me that Saint Guinefort was a dog . . . As to the legend of the child and the snake, I also found it everywhere, and in the same form, albeit with a few variations. Some would have it that, in this place that was already as wooded as it is today, there stood a woodcutter's modest cabin. When he set out to work, he would leave his child in the care of Guinefort, his dog. One day, a snake got into the cabin and made its way towards the child's cradle; the dog halted it and killed it. The woodcutter, reentering his house, saw that the animal's mouth was covered in blood. He believed that it had devoured his child and, like the lord of whom Stephen of Bourbon speaks, he looked no further into the matter but murdered the dog with his axe. The same regret was then expressed in the same fashion, etc.
>
> According to others, the place was then cultivated by some young farmers. The farmer's wife, not wanting to leave her child alone, took it with her in its cradle and, entrusting it to the care of her dog, left it in the corner of a field. As in the two other narratives, a snake approaches, etc.'[5]

There is no longer any room for doubt. These two versions of the legend of the faithful dog, collected in the vicinity of Saint Guinefort's wood, confirm that Stephen of Bourbon suppressed the superstitious cult of Saint Guinefort in this very spot. They also demonstrate the longevity of oral tradition: in the nineteenth century, the peasants living in this region still handed down the legend of the dog saint whom they revered.

These two versions have been imperfectly recorded by Vayssière, but they merit a brief analysis, nevertheless. The first is reminiscent of the simplified versions which I placed within the third group of narratives, for neither the mother nor the nurse is mentioned. The second resembles narrative N7, in which the cradle is not, as in the other narratives in the first group, left in the room, but in which the nurses carry it outside and place it at the foot of the wall.

The most remarkable feature of the two nineteenth-century versions is the reduced social status of the two persons involved. Does it not reflect a fundamental modification in the social relations of the countryside, from the seigneurial system of the Ancien Régime to the peasantry of the post-revolutionary period?

In interpreting Stephen of Bourbon's *exemplum*, we ought therefore to respect certain limits, for, in spite of the obvious continuity of ways of life, the social condition of nineteenth-century peasants was not that of their thirteenth-century ancestors. The peasant narrative transmitted by Stephen of Bourbon has to be considered in terms of a specific, and historically situated, social relation.

Vayssière's 1879 account contradicts Curé Dufournet's 1826 letter regarding the crucial question of the saint's identity. According to the letter, the statuettes that the mendicant dressed as saints were certainly human in form. But the curé being unaware of Stephen of Bourbon's *exemplum*, had not questioned his flock sufficiently closely to discover if they also revered a dog. Once the medieval text had been published, however, it raised new questions and revealed a dimension of the cult that had been hidden since the thirteenth century. It is true that Vayssière had also seen a small statue lodged in the wall beside the road, which was 'considered by many to be a representation of Saint Guinefort.' It was clearly a statue of a human form. But Vayssière simply considers it to be 'a very crude piece of sculpture, meant to be taken for an apostle, but having absolutely nothing in common with Saint Guinefort'. Nowhere is it said that this statue was one of those that the mendicant had dressed in 1826. Must one conclude, however, that a representation of the saint in human form, and the legend in which he appears as a dog, are irreconcilable? I have emphasised the ambiguous status of the hero of the legend, placed as he is between men and beasts. This could have so confused the faithful about the saint's identity that, given the logic of folklore, the legend which represented the saint as a dog existed alongside the statue of him in human form. But Vayssière, given his rationalist bent, could not accept such ambiguities. Since oral tradition went on asserting that Saint Guinefort was a dog, the statue, in spite of the peasants' own considered opinion, must represent some apostle or other.

Vayssière had his own reasons for maintaining so forcefully that the peasants of the Dombes, right up to the end of the nineteenth century, continued to revere a saint who was actually a dog. The foreword to his study sheds some light on his scientific and ideological presuppositions:

Were I to write a history of superstition in the *département* of Ain, on one side I should range all those superstitions that are of a religious nature; on the other I should place all those that were not of such a nature. The second category would, for instance, include belief in witches, the use of formulae and cabbalistic signs in order to check or prevent various illnesses, etc. I should subdivide the second, studying first those superstitions which may be confused with catholic beliefs, and then purely idolatrous beliefs and superstitions. It is in this latter subdivision that I should range the cult of Saint Guinefort.

This attempt at conceptualisation is interesting, even if it culminates in a typology that we would question today, i.e., on the one hand, magic, which would simply comprise acts, and religion on the other. Only in the latter category would 'acts' refer to a system of representations. Among the religious superstitions, some fall under the clerical category of 'improper worship of the true God', or popular distortions of the official religion. Others testify to the persistence of a pre-Christian paganism, entailing the adoration of idols. This is how Vayssière defines the cult of Saint Guinefort (in spite of the title 'Saint', which nevertheless refers to catholicism), since it demonstrates the perennial nature of an idolatrous cult addressed to an animal. This conclusion does not seem to have shocked Vayssière too much, for it is not without some satisfaction that he records that the age-old attempts of the Church to Christianise the countryside had enjoyed a very limited success. One can discern here, in spite of his reticence, the lay spirit that prevailed at the start of the Third Republic. But the catholic counter-offensive was not long in coming!

In 1886, Abbé Delaigue, the chaplain of the hospice at Châtillon-sur-Chalaronne, also published a small work on the 'Pilgrimage of Saint Guinefort'. Without actually mentioning Vayssière, the abbé quotes several passages from his work in order to refute them. He begins with an almost Shakespearean question:

> Those who follow this pilgrimage declare and assert that they go to invoke Saint Guinefort on behalf of their sick children and, since they alone know their real intentions, one must, it seems take them at their word. Some authors, however, no doubt endowed with a talent for reading people's consciences, accuse them of going to the wood at Sandrans, and making their prayers to a dog, and base this accusation on the authority of an old legend. Whom should one believe? In other words, is this Guinefort a *saint* or is he a *dog*? This is the question that must be settled.[6]

He does not hesitate over which answer to give. He marshals a host of arguments to counter 'the scoffing of the free thinkers'. First, the story of the faithful dog is only a 'fabliau which people tell' and not a true history. Admittedly, 'Father Bourbon was a Dominican monk and the province's inquisitor; in both capacities he deserves some respect.' But if he believed this story, and many others as well, along with all the others which he records 'from hearsay' in his treatise, 'one can only conclude that he was remarkably credulous and that people took advantage of his simplicity to laugh at his expense'. And if, of all the equally incredible stories that he has recorded, the free thinkers only recall this one, it is because it gives them the opportunity 'to ridicule piety and religion'.

Secondly, if Stephen of Bourbon did 'in the end', as he himself acknowledges, encounter this legend, it was only after many investigations. Which only went to prove that the legend of the dog was 'unknown to the public', and that a practical joker slipped it to him in order 'to make fun of his simplicity'.

Thirdly, a castle could never have stood on this spot. Moreover, when the *villa* of Clerdan was built, this site was passed over in favour of one nearby, which was 'higher, more extensive, more open and more pleasant'.

Fourthly, 'an advocate of the legend' (i.e., Vayssière) had himself admitted that a statue, lodged in the wall of a house and probably representing an apostle, was said to be Saint Guinefort. The house had since been destroyed, but the abbé questioned the former owner quite closely about it. He concluded that this statue must actually have been in the wood up until the Revolution. He had also heard tell of the mendicant denounced by Curé Dufournet in 1826, but the crude statue which the former used to clothe in rags could not have been the original one from the wood:

> A certain Morel, who lived at Clerdan farm, some thirty years ago, confirmed that there was a statue in Saint Guinefort's wood, and that a wretch had built a cabin there, and that the late Comte de la Rochette had him remove the statue. This latter is not the same as the one we were speaking of before.[7]

The statue which interested Abbé Delaigue was, to his mind, the original cult object that had been in the wood. It had the virtue of being the oldest, and above all, of being easily identified: 'It represents Saint Guinefort in the guise of an Apostle *or* Bishop.' Vayssière had not said as much, but Abbé Delaigue, who was familiar with Saint Millefort or Guinefort of Picardy and Normandy, had no doubts on the subject. For him, they were one and the same saint.

Hence his final argument, which went as follows. Neither in Picardy, nor in Normandy, nor even at Béreins in the Dombes, was Saint Guinefort venerated as a dog. Everywhere, with all due respect to the free thinkers, he was represented as a man.

Things are much the same at Sandrans. The abbé cites the deed executed in 1632, which mentions 'the *hermitures* in which the chapels of Saint Guy le Fort formerly stood', and which represents them as being a series of flimsy constructions comprising a chapel and a hermit's house. And he concludes, forgetting Stephen of Bourbon's testimony a little too quickly: 'It is therefore to a chapel dedicated to Saint Guinefort, and not to the tomb of a dog, that the pilgrimage owes its origin.'

So much for the saint's cult, which has thus been reintegrated into orthodoxy, to the great confusion of the free thinkers. But what of the rite in which the mothers bore their sick children to the place, deposited swaddling-clothes on the bushes, and knotted together branches so as to unknot the sickly limbs? Were these practices supernatural, 'in other words, should one attribute to them a supernatural effect'? Abbé Delaigue asked the pilgrims what their gestures meant, and their answers, although vague, satisfied him: 'I don't know', 'we've always done it like this', 'it is to mark the fact that a child has weak or knotted limbs, and that one desires Saint Guinefort to strengthen or to unknot them'. He also notes that these practices are not considered crucial in causing the saint to take action, since some who visit this place of pilgrimage are wise enough to refrain from these gestures. As for the others, he finishes on a tolerant note: 'When seen in this light, this practice would seem to be an enacted prayer rather than a superstitious act.' Was this the opinion of just one man, or were people in general slowly coming to this conclusion? It certainly contrasts with the criticisms that Curé Dufournet makes of his flock's 'misunderstood religion'. He was, admittedly, mainly concerned with the individual strategies of a mendicant. But not all the clergy shared Abbé Delaigue's opinion, for, once he had refuted the 'free thinkers'' arguments, he also fought on another front, and sought to combat the intolerance of certain priests: 'Some curés – I could name at least two – considered themselves obliged to preach, upon several occasions, against the pilgrimage.' For an ineffectual and unjust suppression, Abbé Delaigue proposed that one substitute the solution that the church held in reserve for just such occasions. One ought, he argued, to build a church upon this spot, whereupon the cult of Saint Guinefort would gain richer, more plentiful, and more sheltered *ex-votos*. This was the solution proposed in 1826 by an obscure mendicant, and the idea may well have caused the Bishop of Belley to smile. But the person who suggested this was unfortunately nothing but a mendicant living in the woods! We do not know why Abbé Delaigue did not, some sixty years later, carry out his project. The final phase of the cult of Saint Guinefort in Sandrans wood would then undoubtedly have been quite different.

In 1886 Baron Raverat published his account of his travels, entitled *De Lyon à Châtillon-sur-Chalaronne, par Marlieux et le chemin de fer à voie étroite*. The baron was not primarily concerned, as Abbé Delaigue had been the previous year, with defending and providing examples of catholic orthodoxy. His faith lay, rather, in technical progress. He began by painting a somewhat sombre picture of the agricultural, demographic and sanitary situation in the Dombes. He then anticipated the crucial changes that the completed Lyons–Bourg railway line, which Châtillon had awaited since 1879, would bring to this region. The train was also a means of discovering historical and picturesque sites, such as the 'famous pilgrimage of Saint Guinefort', along which the baron was taken, from the station at Moulin-des-Champs. His own interpretation is meant as a historical one, whereas the debate between reason and religion, which turned upon the question of Saint Guinefort's identity, had led Vayssière and Abbé Delaigue to abolish history by treating Stephen of Bourbon's text as belonging to the same time-scale as the testimonies of contemporaries. The lack of any historical dimension only made the polemic fiercer. But this was of no interest to the baron, who was a partisan of progress, and an evolutionist concerned to observe the alterations in the cult over time. Now, if the cult of the dog had existed, it belonged (according to the baron) to the past. Priests and free thinkers were thus both sent packing. The Gauls were held to be behind the cult:

> It would, it seems to me, be a facinating study to try and discover the origin of this form of devotion. The serpent, the dog, the fauns, the wolf, the old witch, the immersion in the stream, and above all the pins stuck in the tree-trunks, this entire staging seems to me to belong to the customs and mythology of the Gauls, our ancestors. For we know that they celebrated their ceremonies beside gushing waters, under cover of darkest night, in the mysterious shadows of the forest, in a sacred *lucus*. . .[8]

In Stephen of Bourbon's time, it was still a dog that was worshipped. But little by little, 'popular imagination' substituted the cult of Saint Guinefort for the dog Guinefort. The question was not, therefore, with all its polemical overtones, 'Dog *or* saint?' Everyone could agree over the truth, the baron felt, for Guinefort was first a dog and *then* a saint.

Local folklorists were quite familiar with the cult by the turn of the century. Thus A. Vingtrinier visited the site in 1902 and confirmed that the cult, although lacking a chapel and an altar, was very much alive. He also cites Stephen of Bourbon's testimony, and had no doubts that the whole cult was already in existence 'at the time of the druids'.[9] After him, A. Callet, in 1903, and then the famous Mâconnais folklorist, G. Jeanton, in 1921, simply quoted Vingtrinier, without visiting the wood themselves. Around

1930, Dr Le Tessier went there and noted that the pilgrimage had died out 'ten years ago'.[10]

We therefore lack evidence for the first half of the twentieth century, the very period in which the cult disappeared. When, in 1962, and again in 1970, the doctor in Châtillon-sur-Chalaronne, Dr V. Edouard, reopened the case, the cult of Saint Guinefort was nothing more than a memory. It is significant that the last person, so far as Dr Edouard knew, to have gone (around 1940) to this wood, to effect the cure of a child, was its grandmother and not its mother. The mother and the women of her generation, being younger, had undoubtedly already broken free of this form of devotion. In spite of repeated and careful examination of the evidence (1975–76), I have found no sign in the wood that would lead one to suppose that the cult, even in a very secret and marginal way, is still carried on today, for nothing now remains of all that, but a century ago, was clearly visible in the wood (children's clothes hung upon trees, knotted branches, pieces of money thrown upon the earth). Great caution is required, however, when one comes to interrogate the oral tradition in order to recover the legend of the faithful dog, for a large number of local scholars have, for a century or more, used Stephen of Bourbon's *exemplum* in their publications. One of my informants assured me that 'My grandmother told me: it seems that he was a dog!' It is hard to say if this opinion derives from the versions of the legend collected by Vayssière in 1879 or if it was influenced by all the commentaries on the medieval *exemplum*, which have sprung up over the last hundred years or so.

When one considers how numerous the pilgrims were, which is something that the testimonies of the very end of the last century emphasise, the cult's disappearance would seem to have been very sudden, in or after the first world war. It had, until this date, remained very active.

Vayssière maintained that the pilgrims had, in order to get to the heart of the wood, to take a path which is still visible today, and which runs across the Southern slope of the hill. According to Baron Raverat's account, one was supposed to climb the slope backwards. The motives for going on this pilgrimage in the nineteenth century were varied; one might desire to cure swamp fever, or hope, if one were a young girl, to find a husband, or if one were a woman, to restore one's husband's or lover's potency. But the main reason was, as in the thirteenth century, a concern to restore one's children to good health if they were 'ailing', 'feverish', or 'rachitic'. Mothers would tie the branches together in order to 'knot the fever', or to 'unknot' a child's legs if it was slow in learning to walk. It was considered auspicious if the sap happened to weld two branches together. In order to rid the child of its illness, they would leave its shirt, its shoes, or its swaddling-clothes on bushes. A. Vayssière saw 'knotted branches by the thousand', 'a mass of articles of clothing', which suggests that the wood was indeed frequented by a large number of people. The information that he had gathered would seem to suggest that women came from as far afield as the mountains around Lyons and the *département* of Isère. He also drew attention to the presence in the wood of a large number of little crosses of plaited grass, like those that are placed in the fields on 3 May, on the feast of the Invention of the Holy Cross. Before leaving the woods, the women would throw on the ground, or bury, several pieces of money.

Some important features of the pilgrimage that Stephen of Bourbon described may thus still be recognised in the nineteenth century. But there are also crucial differences, for Stephen of Bourbon made no reference to knotted branches, nor to plaited crosses of grass, nor to gifts of pieces of money. Conversely, in the nineteenth century, people were no longer immersed in the Chalaronne, even though the path that the women took leads straight to the river. If, finally, the thirteenth-century rite was meant to rid one of a changeling, and to recover the stolen child, the nineteenth-century one only involved a cure, and not a substitution. European folklore in the nineteenth century does, however, suggest a belief in changelings.

It is no simple matter to interpret these differences, for once again we have to do with observations that are uneven in quality. The rite's alteration may well be more apparent than real, and the most remarkable feature of this cult is the perennial nature of the ritual forms, inscribed as they are in an unchanging space.

Stephen of Bourbon also emphasised the part played by a *vetula* in assisting and guiding the mothers during the rite. Tradition may have required that some person playing such a role be associated with the place. The mendicant mentioned in 1826 also claimed to know about the origins of the cult, and for a small reward would offer his services to pilgrims. At any rate, he resided in the wood, whereas the witch in the thirteenth century came from a *castrum* a league or so distant. Now, my own fieldwork brought to light a 'witch', similar to the *vetula* in the *exemplum*, who had played a comparable role around 1930. She lived in Châtillon-sur-Chalaronne, 'a league or so distant' from Saint Guinefort's wood.

I questioned a dozen or so people from Châtillon, aged from fifty to ninety, men and women, all of whom had a very clear memory of her. People called her 'la Fanchette Gadin'. No one doubted that this was her real name, but at the same time each person gave some explanation of the etymology: under her dress 'she wore pebbles (*gadins*), so that the devil would not bear her off. But if he had carried her off, he would have brought her back the next morning, she was that ugly.' There was another explanation too: she threw stones at the boys who mocked her ('the girls were afraid of her'). She lived at Châtillon, in a hut at the foot of the castle, in a district whose inhabitants were all 'much the same'. There was 'Père Rol', for instance, whom one sought out when there was a case of worms. She was also compared to Françoise Parcoret, 'who was the same sort of person'. My informants were unanimous in asserting that she lived alone, and that she had never married. Perhaps she had a nephew who lived elsewhere. Apparently she died around 1930, in the almshouse at Châtillon.

She was blind in one eye, and 'as ugly as sin'. Some remember her to have been tall, others see her as small and dumpy. Apart from her dress that was weighted with stones, she wore a headdress with white fringes. She would hoard and live off cress and dandelion. She pushed a pram in front of her, and on Mondays she would go out begging, for 'she had her houses'. The former preceptor, for instance, would give her ten centimes. She cast spells, but spared those who gave her meat. She also paid a visit to the grandmother of one of my informants, whom she asked 'to pick up her stitches' (for she knitted a great deal, though blind in one eye). In summer, she offered 'some small yellow flowers from Saint Roch, to my grandmother, as a precaution against fire'. She spent a large part of her time in the cemetery ('when she was missing, one would find her in the cemetery'), where she would weed the graves. She also went to church, 'but only for others', for she would light candles on request for a small fee. On Saturday she said novenas for livestock and for people. But, above all, she went on 'journeys', going on foot to the pilgrimage sites in the region, but always for other people and on payment of a small fee. If a child had whooping-cough she would visit the church bells at Neuville. She went to Notre-Dame-de-Beaumont in order 'to curl the children's hair', and to Saint-Philomène-d'Ars 'for worms'. When young 'she had seen the curé at Ars, who had refused her confession because she wanted to go dancing. He guessed all.' One of the local pilgrimages upon which she was wont to go was that of Saint Guinefort. Such women, whose task it was to carry out 'substitute' pilgrimages, were often the repositories of oral traditions,[11] but I did not hear of la Fanchette Gadin knowing or telling the legend of the faithful dog. She carried pieces of money given to her by the children's parents, and she made vows for their cure. Several informants summed up the very strong impression that la Fanchette Gadin had made upon them as follows: 'She was a real character!'

Since she died at the almshouse in Châtillon, where Dr Edouard remembered having cared for her, I had hoped to find a medical file on her. But I looked in vain, because at that time the institution in question did not yet hold any card-indexes on its residents. I therefore had to make do with what the State could offer in the way of completing, checking, and perhaps shedding some light on my oral sources. My first perusal of the registers between 1920 and 1940 yielded no 'Fanchette Gadin'. But, upon quoting to my informants some names close to the one that they had attributed to her, we soon discovered that she was actually called Françoise Gudin. It was then a simple matter to reconstruct her biography.

Françoise Tremblay, called Gudin, was born on 9 January 1848, and died at the Châtillon almshouse on 23 November 1936. Her father, Antoine Tremblay, called Gudin (1802–47), son of a journeyman, was a ropemaker at Châtillon. In 1845 he married a journeywoman from Châtillon, Marie-Denise Chambard (1812–90), and upon this occasion acknowledged the son that she had had by him seven years before, Michel Chambard. A year after their marriage, in 1846, they had a second child, Rose Tremblay, called Gudin, who was later to marry, follow the profession of laundry-woman, and die in 1879. Eighteen months after Rose, Françoise (the 'Fanchette Gadin' of our story) was born, some two months after the death of her father. At the age of twenty-nine, a journeywoman and unmarried, she brought into the world a still-born boy (3 May 1877). In 1883, at the age of thirty-five, she married a fifty-four-year-old widower, Jean-Marie Ducotté (1829–1910), described as a mason on the marriage certificate, but simply as a journeyman on the death certificate. The couple were childless. Widowed in 1910, Françoise Gudin, widow Ducotté, lived henceforth on her own, since her sister and mother had long since died. She remained without any family for a further twenty-six years, until her death at the age of eighty-eight. People forgot that she had been married for twenty-seven years. The nephew to whom they sometimes referred may have been a son of her sister Rose, or it may have been her own brother, Michel Chambard.

It is of real interest to compare this woman's official biography with the memories that she left behind her. Coming from a very modest background (her people were mainly journeymen), it is fair to say that, from her birth onwards, she lost whatever slight opportunities she had had. Born in the difficult years of 1846–8, her mother having been left with a ten-year old boy and two babies, she was also one of those 'posthumous children' who are thought to be singled out by fate, and therefore endowed with therapeutic powers for the rest of their lives. There is undoubtedly some connection between the peculiar nature of her birth and her subsequent role in healing pilgrimages. Then there was her still-born child, and after a series of difficulties that it is none too hard to imagine, a late marriage. Then widowhood, poverty, and solitude, and an infirmity which undoubtedly does much to explain the 'evil eye' for which she was feared. We know how important a part she played in the community from the precise and full nature of the memories she left behind her. It is only fitting that there should be some other trace of her besides the dry formulae of the State, for this is indeed all that now remains. Her grave, which was in the cemetery at Châtillon-sur-Chalaronne, was flattened in 1974.

The case of Fanchette Gadin may perhaps help us to understand who the *vetula* denounced by Stephen of Bourbon may have been, i.e., nothing more and nothing less than an old woman having, like Fanchette Gadin, a special relationship with death, illness and the devil, and with plants and religious matters. Both, for all their miseries, happened moreover to have had a similar fortune in that they were born, one a little before, and one a little after, a great witch-hunter had visited the area.

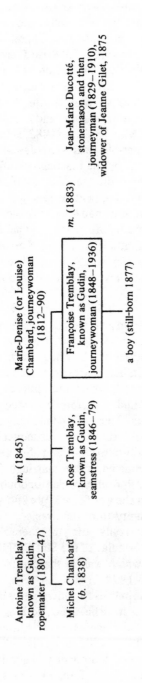

Table 5 'Fanchette Gadin': family tree

9

DOG AND SAINT

When, in 1879, A. Vayssière had the good fortune to discover that the legend of the dog had not been forgotten by the pilgrims in the wood at Sandrans, he enquired after the name of the holy dog:

> All those whom I approached told me that Saint Guinefort was a dog. Some believe that his master named him thus because he never stopped wagging his tail; others suppose that the expression 'Guignefort' was meant as an encouragement.

According to this 'popular etymology', the knight had called his dog 'Guignefort' because it 'winked' (*guigner*), i.e., made little signs whilst wagging its tail. The dog had therefore become a saint because the pilgrims took the movements of its tail to mean that their prayers had been favourably received. The statue of Saint Blaise at Torcieu was likewise said to 'wink' his eye at young girls who wanted a husband, this wink signifying that their wishes would come true.[1]

In a yet more realistic vein, the peasants of Sandrans used to say that the movement of the tail of the holy dog Guignefort was taken as a sign of encouragement by men whose virility was troubling them.

The history of the French language does not contradict these explanations, for in Old French just as in modern *patois*, *guigner* means 1. to make a sign, 2. to make a sign with the eye, 3. to shake, and therefore where a dog was concerned, to make a sign by shaking or wagging one's tail. The peasants questioned by Stephen of Bourbon could have commented upon Saint Guinefort's name in much the same terms as those of the nineteenth century did. It is worth bearing in mind, on the other hand, that the derivative, *guignon*, 'misfortune', associated with the idea of the evil eye, is not encountered before 1609, and that the modern French expression *avoir la guigne* ('to have bad luck') did not occur before 1821. We cannot therefore read the same significance into the thirteenth-century document.[2]

There is another document, however, from the beginning of the thirteenth century, which confirms the 'popular etymology' quoted above. An *exemplum* of Jacques de Vitry begins as follows:

> I have heard that in France there was a demon that spoke and practised the art of divination through the mouth of a demoniac, who thus divulged numerous secrets, and everyone was of the

opinion that he did not lie. A man having come one day to ask him some questions, Guinehochet (for this is what the demon called himself) told the truth about everything. . .[3]

The prefix and suffix of this demon's name mean almost the same thing, for *hochet* derives from the verb *hochier*, to shake, to move or to tremble. Hence the secondary meaning, 'to play at dice, or at heads or tails', and the noun *hochet*, which from this period on refers to a child's game.[4] The pleonasm 'Guinehochet' evokes both the demoniac's trembling and the power of the demon to 'signify' the true and the false. Likewise, Saint Guinefort's name could have been associated with the legend of a greyhound that was unjustly killed, and whom the peasants would entreat to receive their requests with a favourable eye.

Other phonetic associations could well have played some part in this. Baron Raverat, and more recently, Dr Edouard reckoned that the phonetic resemblance between the *patois* words *lou tsin* (i.e., *le chien*, 'the dog') and *lou tsaint* (*le saint*, 'the saint') had contributed to the sanctification of the dog Guignefort. There are regions in which these two terms are actually the object of a pun, particularly in the case of Saint Roch, and the dog that is his attribute: 'Saint Roch et sin tchin', people say in the Pas-de-Calais. The pun probably occurs in the case of Saint Guinefort also.[5]

Besides, even if the greyhound in the legend has no name, it is reasonable to ask whether the name 'Guinefort' was a dog's name in the twelfth or thirteenth century, for this would have facilitated the assimilation of the saint to the dog. There are, in fact, similar names (formed with the same suffix, *fort*) given in French medieval literature to several animals that were cherished by their masters. Florence de Rome's horse (in the first quarter of the thirteenth century) was called Brunfort, and Ogier of Denmark's (twelfth century) Broiefort. It seems to have been because he was so remarkably strong, and because his neighing was so vigorous, that he was called by this name.[6] Jacques de Fouilloux's treatise on venery also mentions a dog called Tirefort.[7] But, so far as I know, no romance or medieval treatise on dogs mentions a dog called Guinefort. It is not a dog's name.

There is one case which I ought, however, to mention, for it too concerns a greyhound. In the First Continuation of Chrétien de Troyes's *Perceval*, Carados learns that his true father is not the husband of his mother Ysave, but the magician Eliaurès, with whom she had committed the sin of adultery. In order to take revenge upon Eliaurès, Carados forces him to couple with a *lisse*, i.e., a greyhound bitch, with a sow and with a mare. Each of these female animals lets drop a little one, which receives a name. The piglet is called Tortain, the colt Lorigal and the young greyhound Guinalot:

> Et de la lisse od cui coucha
> Un waignon concheü en a

Qui fu apelez Guinalot
Si estoit frères Caradot.[8]
(The greyhound with which he coupled
conceived a dog
which was called Guinalot;
It was brother to Carados.)

The name of this young greyhound is not dissimilar to 'Guinefort'. Even though we lack the complete name, does the prefix perhaps have some link with the animal that concerns us? It is worth noting that, in Old French, an admittedly rare form of the verb *graigner* ('to growl', 'to threaten', 'to bite') is *guinier*. This form would seem to occur both in 'Guinefort' and in 'Guinalot'; it is also reminiscent of the hostile attitude of the greyhound towards the serpent. Béroul's *Tristan* quotes it in a fairly eloquent manner:

[Li chiens] mis estoit a grant frëor
Quant il ne voiet son seignor
Ne vout mengier ne pain ne past
Ne nule rien qu'en lui donast;
Guignout et si feroit du pié,
Des viz lermant. Deus! quel pitié
Faisait a mainte gent li chiens![9]

(The dog was overcome by a terrible fear
When he could no longer see his master.
He would eat neither bread nor bran
Nor anything that was put before him.
He would growl and scratch with his paws
With tears upon his face. God! What pity
This dog inspired in so many people.)

This verb *guigner*, which differs from the first form, may be compared with a modern form which derives from it, and which has been noted by folklorists, i.e., *dégueniller*, which means, where a dog is concerned, to throw oneself upon a man or an animal, bite them, and tear them apart with one's bare teeth.[10]

All the hypotheses advanced so far lay some emphasis on the phonetic and semantic associations which constitute what is usually called 'popular etymology'. But 'scientific etymology' ought not to be neglected either. What is the scientific etymology of the name 'Guinefort'?

Guinefort is a person's name, whose construction, inasmuch as it links a root with a suffix, implies a Germanic origin. The root *guini-* (or *wini-*) is found in a large number of names of Germanic persons, such as Guinifredus (Winifrid), which is encountered in the Lombardy region.[11] It is worth noting that numerous saints have names of this kind, for instance, Saint Winebaud, Saint Winifride, and above all Saint Winifrid, better known as

Saint Boniface (*c.* 680–754). The Latin version of this name indicates what its root, *wini-*, must mean. This implies the notions of gain, prosperity, and friendship, and it reappears in the modern German verb *gewinnen*, 'to win', and in the noun *Wünsch*, 'a wish'.

The origin of this name probably explains why it should have been attributed to a legendary Lombard saint, Saint Guinefort of Pavia. But it is equally clear that it could not have been this etymology that caused the peasants of the Dombes, in the twelfth to thirteenth centuries, to associate the saint's name with the greyhound of the legend.

It is with some relief that I bring my study of Saint Guinefort's name to a halt here, for in the field of onomastics and the applied etymology of folklore, misconceptions have been so common, even up to very recently, that it would seem best not to transgress the bounds of common sense by pursuing it any further.

We have shown that there was undoubtedly a historical link between the two cult sites, at Pavia and at Sandrans, and that the diffusion of the Pavia cult caused the saint's name, as well as his status as martyr, to be known at Sandrans. A number of phonetic and semantic connections would also seem to have led to an association between the memory of Saint Guinefort the martyr and the legend of the faithful greyhound that had been unjustly killed by its master.

All that the two cult sites would seem to have in common is a saint's name, and a martyr's and holy healer's reputations. Yet the nature of the knight's dog, on the one hand, and the date of the saint's feast day (22 August), on the other, suggest that there may well have been a fundamental link between the clerical cult at Pavia and the folk cult at Sandrans.

In my analysis of the cult of Saint Guinefort, I have chosen to emphasise the dates of the saints' feast days. This emphasis may in general be justified by the importance of calendar cycles in folk culture. Moreover, in the case of Saint Guinefort, the formal differences in the cult from place to place are themselves proof enough of the significance of the calendar. For at Pavia, where Saint Guinefort is a man, he is celebrated on 22 August, whereas at Sandrans, where he is a dog, he is honoured throughout the year.

Saint Guinefort is not the only saint to have been represented as a dog, for Saint Christopher was also. According to the most ancient versions of his legend, which are Eastern in origin, he was a giant with a dog's head. Until the time at which he was converted to Christ, he devoured men. Jacques de Voragine said that he was of Chananean origin, i.e., in etymological terms, that he came from the land of the dogs. There are Greek traditions according to which he comes from Lycopolis and Lycia respectively, the town and the country of wolves, or from Cynopolis or Cynopolitania, the town and the country of dogs. Iconographic representations include his dog's head and his saint's halo within the same picture. This is a particularly Byzantine

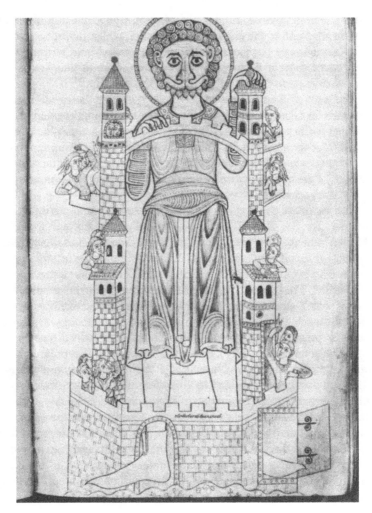

7 A cynocephalous Saint Christopher, from a twelfth-century Martyrology (Hist. fol. 415, fol. 50ʳ), Stuttgart, Landesbibliothek

tradition, but it also occurs in the West, as in a book of martyrs of the second half of the twelfth century[12] (Illustration 7).

Now, as P. Saintyves[13] has shown, the Byzantine church celebrated Saint Christopher on 9 May, while the medieval Christian church celebrated him on 25 July. On this latter date, the Coptic church celebrated Saint Mercury, who has much in common with Saint Christopher. These two dates correspond respectively to the setting of the dog-star (Sirius) and to its rising in the constellation Canis major. These Christian festivals would seem to have 'succeeded' pagan festivals which took place on the same dates, and with a similar symbolism. Thus in May, in Egypt, the cult of Anubis, the dog-headed god of the dead, was celebrated, whilst in Greece, on 25 July, the *Kunophontes* (or massacre of dogs) ceremony was performed. On the very same date, in Rome, when the waters were at their lowest, all red-haired dogs were sacrificed to the goddess Furrina.[14]

The cult of Saint Christopher clearly did not 'succeed' these pagan festivals in a literal sense, for the Christian religious system to which it belongs is far too dissimilar for one to assert that a particular saint was substituted for a pagan god. There is, nevertheless, a striking continuity, and one that serves to prove how important the observation of the stars, and the effects of their conjunctions, may be in the religious representations of traditional societies.

The ascent of the dog-star (Sirius) heralds a crucial period of the year, namely, the dog-days. This is a period of great heat and drought in the Mediterranean, and ever since classical times it has been thought to encourage epidemics and rabies.[15] This accounts for a large part of the symbolism which is associated with Saint Christopher at the beginning of this period. The theme of the dog clearly derives from this tradition, as does that of water, since the saint enabled the infant Christ to cross the river, and the vegetation theme likewise (for its struggles in the dog-days against the sun's oppressive heat); when Saint Christopher arrived on the opposite bank, he planted his staff in the earth, whereupon it sprouted once again, was covered in flowers and bore fruit. P. Saintyves compared this aspect of the legend with the rites for the Invention of the Holy Cross, which took place in Europe at the beginning of May, upon the same day as the feast of Saint Christopher is celebrated in the Greek Orthodox church. Little crosses of plaited grass were placed in the fields in order to obtain good harvests, and the peasants would pick them up again at harvest time. Sometimes people would also place images of serpents at the foot of the statue of Saint Christopher 'and his hagiographers did not know how to account for their presence, but supposed that it might be because of their beneficial power'.

The dog-days, which begin with the feast of Saint Christopher on 25 July, finish when Sirius sets once more in Canis major on 24 August. Now this date, give or take a day or two, is also the feast of Saint Guinefort at Pavia, a martyr who was pierced with arrows, who was invoked against the plague, and therefore associated in litanies with Saint Christopher and Saint Roch. Admittedly, the Saint Guinefort who was at Pavia had no dog as his attribute (he simply had the martyr's palm and the *miles*'s sword), and was not, *a fortiori*, represented as a dog. Nor does any dog feature in his legend, whereas at Sandrans pilgrims conceived of Saint Guinefort as a greyhound and more generally, in the nineteenth century, as a dog.

Numerous saints who have a dog as their attribute, or who are themselves compared symbolically with dogs, have their feasts between 25 July and 24 August, the dates which open and close the dog-days.

Admittedly, all the saints honoured in July and August are not represented as being in the company of a dog. This is particularly the case with those saints with whom Saint Guinefort has sometimes been confused (with the sole exception of Saint Guy), namely, Saint Wilgeforte (20 July), Saint Cucuphas (25 July), or with whom he has been associated, at Puy for example. Conversely, not all the saints associated with a dog have feasts during this period. Thus, Saint Hubert, the patron saint of hunters, invoked against rabies, is honoured on 3 November. But no other part of the year has so great a concentration of saints who are represented as being in the company of a dog.[16] Suppose we consider the widest possible definition of this period, i.e., from 3 or 7 May (the first setting of Sirius) to 24 August (the second setting of Sirius), when the dog-days, which begin with the rising of the star in the constellation of the dog, are ended. This period contains the following saints represented as being in the company of a dog, in this order:

On 22 May, Saint Quiterie (or Guiteria), virgin and martyr, invoked in Spain and Gascony against rabid dogs.

On 15 June, Saint Guy (Vitus), martyr, a native of Lucania or of Sicily, subsequently invoked in North Italy and then in Northern Europe, against epilepsy ('Saint Guy's or Saint Vitus's dance'), and against the bites of dogs, wolves and snakes. One has all the more reason to compare him to Saint Guinefort, in fact, in that the hermitage at Tournus, in the seventeenth century was attributed to one (Saint Guy le Fort) or the other of the two saints. One clearly cannot account for the confusion between saints in terms of the resemblance between their names. The feast's date, function and mode of representation are equally crucial.

On 4 July, Saint Ulrich, Bishop of Augsbourg (d. 973), was held to offer protection against the bite of rabid dogs.

During the dog-days themselves, and after the festival of Saint Christopher, we encounter:

On 4 August, Saint Dominic, founder of the Dominican order, or, thanks to the pun that his name inspired, of the 'dogs of the lord' (*domini canes*). The saint himself had been identified with a dog:

> Before his birth, his mother saw herself in a dream with a little dog at her breast; it had a lighted torch in its mouth, with which it lit up the whole universe. When she had given birth to little Dominic, a lady who had lifted him up to the sacred baptismal font thought that she saw upon his forehead a brilliant star illuminating the whole earth.

We have here an explicit reference to the symbolism of the stars, even if the star itself is not named. The torch's flames evoke the symbolism of the dog-days, an impression that is reinforced by the extreme importance accorded to the themes of fire and water in the subsequent legend of the saint. He was thought to save those who were in danger of drowning, and to hold off the rain wherever he went. We find that, in other places, his writings were spared by the fire (the miracle of Montreal) and, in order to convert the heretical matrons of Fanjeaux, Saint Dominic caused the devil to leap around in front of them, in the guise of a terrifying cat 'which had the proportions of a big dog, with huge, flaming eyes'.[17]

Saint Roch, who is held to offer even greater protection against the plague than Saint Christopher and Saint Guinefort, is honoured on 16 August. Having himself fallen victim to the plague, he was miraculously cured by water from a spring. A hunting dog, unbeknown to his master, brought him bread to eat. Upon following the animal and discovering the saint, this knight was converted to Christianity.

Saint Bernard of Clairvaux, whom his mother saw before his birth, and in a dream, in the form of a dog, is honoured on 20 August. This tradition, mentioned in the very first *Life* of the saint, has much in common with the legend of Saint Dominic:

> Being pregnant with Bernard, her third son, she [his mother] had a dream which foretold the future. She saw at her breast a little white dog, which had a completely red back, and which was barking. She told of this dream to a man of God, who answered her in a prophetic manner: 'You shall be the mother of a fine little dog, which is destined to be the guardian of the house of God; he shall bay at the enemies of the faith, for he shall be a distinguished preacher, who will cure many people through the virtues of his tongue.[18]

This last remark alludes to the healing properties traditionally attributed to the tongues of dogs. Thus, for instance, Hildegard of Bingen says that 'The heat of a dog's tongue will cure wounds and ulcers.'

Other episodes in Saint Bernard's life are also worth citing:

> Bernard had once allowed his eyes to linger over a woman, whereupon he blushed and inflicted a very cruel retribution upon his own body, for he cast himself into a pond whose water was frozen. He remained there until almost frozen stiff and, through God's grace, extinguished all his desire for the pleasures of the flesh.

After this episode, and after two women had tried in vain to seduce him, he decided to enter a monastery: 'Thinking that it is not safe to dwell with a serpent, he decided to take flight, and thenceforth resolved to enter the Cistercian order.'

Finally, on 22 August, the very same day upon which Saint Guinefort is honoured at Pavia, the feast of Saint Dominic of Sora (or Foligno), who died in 1031, is celebrated at Villalago, in the Abruzzi, and at Sora, in Southern Latium.[19] The official date, in the liturgy, for this saint's feast, is 22 January. But the popular festivals, which have for long been associated with his name in Latium, Umbria, and the Abruzzi, have always been held in May, at the earliest, and most often in August, and on the 22nd in particular. The saint is believed to have the power to free the lands of the community of the snakes which infest it, and to chase away wolves. At Cocullo, a tooth of the saint is piously preserved, for it offers protection against snake-bites. Two remarkable rituals take place upon the occasion of this saint's feast day. The pilgrims entwine snakes, which have been captured during the preceding days, around the processional statue, and offer them to the saint in return for his protection. A *sacra rappresentazione* also takes place, during which a man disguised as a wolf pretends to steal a baby, which is inevitably saved by the saint's timely intervention.

The hagiographies provide us with further evidence and testimony regarding medieval representations of the dog-days. Thus, for the thirteenth-century hagiographer Vincent of Beauvais:

> The dog-star, also known as Sirius, is in the middle of the sky during the summer months, and as the sun climbs towards it, its heat, added to that of the sun, is doubled, and bodies are dissolved and go up in smoke . . . It is called 'dog' because it afflicts bodies with illness, or on account of the heat of the flame which it emits. . . That dogs are most vulnerable to rabies during this part of the year is indisputable. . .[20]

He is here reiterating some of Pliny's conclusions, as transmitted by Isidore of Seville. Thirteenth-century astronomers or doctors, such as Arnaud de Villeneuve or Gilbert of England, say much the same.[21]

References to the dog-days are much less frequent in the French medieval literature. Thus, Christine de Pisan simply deplores 'the burning and excessive heat of the dog-days of summertime'.[22]

Finally, there is much to be learned from the material culture of the period. Thus, the firedogs which decorate fireplaces may perhaps derive their name, which is first attested in 1287, from the dogs' heads which were placed beside the hearth fire.[23]

Recent oral evidence is much more specific. Thus, in contemporary French folklore, the dog-days are hedged around with the most detailed prescriptions. One should not bathe for fear of catching a chill, and so as not to suffer from sunstroke, because the waters are too stagnant, or 'because the blood is too agitated during the hot season'.[24] In Germany, people were recommended not to marry during the *Hundstage* (dog-days), and not to undergo bleeding. The prohibition of bleeding was justified by the fact that too much overheated blood would gush forth, and that the sick person's life would thereby be endangered. In England, a sick woman explained it as follows: 'It's the dog-star's fault. Things will not improve until Saturday, until the dog-days are over. It is a bad star.[25] The dog-days did, however, have a positive aspect, in that they were thought to favour hunting.[26]

Local folklore adds something to our knowledge of the representations which are associated with the dog-days. North of Burgundy and as far as the Meuse and the Moselle, the meal served at the close of hay-making and harvest was 'kill-dog'. In Brie, people talk of 'making the dog of August', or of 'making the harvest dog', and in Franche-Comté they say 'When one wishes to kill one's dog, one calls it *cagne*', a word that derives from the Old French *gaignon*, a dog. This ceremonial meal for the month of August may admittedly be named after other animals (cat, hare, she-donkey, cock etc.) in other parts of the country, or after the kind of meat that happened to be served on that occasion. In the area with which we are concerned here, the only name encountered, even nowadays, is *revolle*, first recorded in the *Compte des Syndics* from Châtillon-sur-Chalaronne in 1449. No satisfactory etymology has been proposed.[27]

I would thus argue that the beliefs associated with the dog-days may well have helped to transfer the name and title of Saint Guinefort, martyr, honoured on 22 August at Pavia, to the legendary greyhound from Sandrans.

A fair number of the themes from the hagiographic legends, beliefs and rites associated with the dog-days recur in the legend and rite of Sandrans, such as we know them from the *exemplum*. Thus, in the legend, there is an opposition between dog, archetypal emblem of the dog-days, and snake. This opposition may be explained in terms of the themes of hot and cold, dry and humid, for snakes are cold, whereas dogs are hot, and snakes are also humid, in that they are closer to the earth. Another significant theme is that of the gushing forth of the blood, which pollutes the greyhound's head and the soil. I ought, finally, to mention the growth of trees, which is reminiscent of the staff of Saint Christopher, 'which puts forth shoots'. If one also takes various parallel narratives into consideration, one may also identify the theme of hunting, so crucial to the two versions of the *Dolopathos* in particular, and also the theme of the rabid dog. Thus, in N7, when the nurses come back down again from the battlements surrounding the town, they find the greyhound baying in the courtyard and believe 'that he was rabid and out of his mind'. One may, nevertheless, object that legend N1 does not specify a time of year, and that if one had to suggest a particular time, a consideration of the other versions would lead one to think of Pentecost or Trinity, of spring at any rate, rather than of summer, the period of the dog-days. It is also in spring that the snake 'goes out'. But it is equally active in summer: 'In the coldest part of the winter, snakes twist themselves into knots which they untie in the summer', says Vincent of Beauvais.

The rite itself is performed by women (who are themselves, like the snake, humid) who bring the fire which burns, and who end up by dipping the child in the cold water of the Chalaronne.

It is still more difficult here to reconcile the evidence with the calendar, for at Sandrans the cult does not take place on 22 August, as at Pavia, but the whole year round. Must one therefore reject this hypothesis utterly? The comparison between the various forms of the cult of Saint Guinefort has shown that its staggering throughout the year was attributable to its folklorisation, for in its ecclesiastical form it was always celebrated at one particular moment in the year. One should, moreover, be on one's guard against giving too schematic a presentation of the evidence, for at Pavia also, Saint Guinefort was and sometimes still is honoured throughout the year, even if, on 22 August, he receives more of the faithful, and more ostentatiously. Conversely, a comparative study of the numerous 'permanent' folk pilgrimages, in Bresse, Dombes and Mâconnais in particular, would demonstrate that the pilgrims are invariably more numerous in the high season, and above all in summer, before the major agricultural tasks begin again. This would very probably also have been the case in the wood of Saint Guinefort.

For a long time now, historians have had to choose between a peremptory assertion about 'historical truths' and silence. Yet certainties often turn out to be fragile, and a hypothesis that is still hardly substantiated may be more fruitful than a 'definitive' conclusion. Let us leave it as follows: the peasants of the Dombes, having learned, doubtless through the Cluniacs, of the name and reputation of Saint Guinefort, assimilated him to the greyhound who, in the legend, had been unjustly killed by his master. A whole range of verbal assonances and semantic connections may be held to account for this association between the greyhound and the saint. Moreover, owing to the date of his feast day, and the powers against the plague that his martyr's arrows symbolised, Saint Guinefort of Pavia was a saint of the dog-days. The peasants of the Dombes may well have accepted him for this reason, identifying him with a martyred dog and dedicating a cult to him, several elements of which appear to be linked to the symbolism of the dog-days.

PART 4

Narrative time, historical time

While the cult described by Stephen of Bourbon involves ritual practices of very ancient provenance, whose 'origins' cannot really be traced, the historian is less at a loss where the legend of the faithful dog and references to Saint Guinefort are concerned. For their history provides us with chronological markers which are so close that we can date their convergence very precisely.

The legend of the faithful dog (if, at any rate, we hold to the diffusion and vulgarisation hypothesis which, in the present case, would seem as probable as that of autocthony) can hardly have been known to the peasants of the Dombes before the twelfth century, especially if we bear in mind that the first recorded version in learned culture appears around 1155. We have no precise date for the cult of Saint Guinefort of Pavia prior to 1082, near Allevard. It is therefore probable that the legend of the dog and memory of the saint converged, along with the rite, between the end of the eleventh and the beginning of the twelfth century, if Stephen of Bourbon was to observe, around 1250, the functioning of a perfectly coherent cultural ensemble. The analysis of the structure of this ensemble does not excuse us, therefore, from the task of tackling the problem of its origin.

The narrative collected by Stephen of Bourbon has a history. Indeed, he himself presents it as the narrative of a history. He describes and explains ('by divine will') the alterations in the countryside and the changes that occurred because of the occupation and use of a particular site. An estate (*terre*) inhabited and dominated by a *castrum* (a knight's castle or a fortified village) must have been abandoned. A wood must quickly have sprung up there, which was then visited by peasants bearing their sick children. This history is presented as the narrative of an abandonment.

An examination of the map reproduced on pp. 128–9 shows how central Saint Guinefort's wood is to it, even today, and reveals also a series of place names of varying ages, which testify to the antiquity of the successive stages of occupation of the site. Cerdun (first mentioned in 1215), to the north of Saint Guinefort's wood, is undoubtedly Gallic in origin (from the name of a man, *Siros*, followed by the suffix -*dunum*, meaning 'fortress'). Romans is a typical Latin place name, while Sandrans is of Germanic origin (from the name of a man, *Sanderad*, with the suffix -*ing*), known since 984. Other place names are more recent; for instance, those which derive from the word *castrum* (Châtillon-sur-Chalaronne, Le Châtelard) or which reproduce a saint's name (Saint Georges-sur-Renom) are characteristic of the feudal epoch.

There are, moreover, several place names which suggest that the nature of the site's occupation had altered. The name of Neuville, mentioned by Stephen of Bourbon, implies a recent foundation. We have evidence of the existence of this parish, which was dependent upon a monastery, from the beginning of the eleventh century.[1] To the North-East of Saint Guinefort's wood, the place name Aux Nemes, from the Latin *nemus*, a wood, refers to a forest covering which, at the time, had perhaps already disappeared. The thirteenth-century name *silva Rimite*, and the seventeenth-century expression *les hermitures*, allude either to a memory of hermitages or, more probably, to lands left fallow.

The countryside of Western Europe was, from the eleventh to the fifteenth century, most deeply marked by three phenomena, namely, land clearances, the establishment of new centres of population, and abandonments. The third contrasts with the other two, but is inseparable from them, for even though it was a period of extensive land clearance, the yet faster exhaustion of newly acquired lands, the search for new territory, and the continuing availability of space all favoured high population mobility and thus allowed forest and fallow to reclaim their own.[2] In many regions, as was the case with the town of Latium studied by Pierre Toubert, *castra* which were quite distinct from previous forms of occupation of the land were established during the tenth, eleventh and twelfth centuries, by lords who fortified them and assembled their men there. This *incastellamento* was accompanied by a complete restructuring of space, of the rural economy, and of political, social and ideological relations. But not all the *castra* built from the tenth to the twelfth century, in the mountains of Latium, survived. Almost as many were abandoned (eighty) as continued (around ninety). The point is that the two processes, far from succeeding each other, were simultaneous. If failures were so common and so sudden it was owing to a bad choice of site, or because it was impossible to draw into an organic whole the fields that would be necessary to sustain a peasant community. A place name or several ruins may bear witness, on a particular site, to the ephemeral existence of a *castrum* that had quickly disappeared. Sometimes, abandonment was partial, and the *castrum* was simply demoted to the rank of *casale*, or large farm. This did not disguise a lord's failure:

> If, in a period of full demographic expansion, a village was reduced to a *casale*, this invariably meant that the lord had failed, that he had been forced to convert it to a more niggardly scale, with all that such a renunciation implies in the way of relinquishment of profits, of powers of command and justice over the men assembled there, and of the possibility of extending the area under cultivation.[3]

As Toubert's book shows, historians are now concentrating upon those abandonments which occurred prior to the better-known *Wüstungen* of the fourteenth and fifteenth centuries, and upon the parallel incidence, in a period of expansion, of the establishment and abandonment of habitats. This emphasis helps to explain the effects of these events upon the organisation and patterning of land. This is why it is necessary to undertake a minute cartographic study of these phenomena, as Walter Janssen's magisterial work on the Eifel demonstrates. Janssen investigates the dismantling of a territory which occurs when secondary centres are created, or, on the other hand, the reconstitution that may occur if it subsumes a neighbouring territory whose centre has been abandoned. In either case, the territory becomes unbalanced and its boundaries ill defined, and these factors, when juxtaposed with all the others (archival information, archaeology, oral tradition), inform us about the history of each community.[4]

The *communes* in the region with which we are concerned here tend to have fields that are regular in shape, e.g., a huge triangle at Châtillon-sur-Chalaronne, a rectangle at Romans, etc. The main village, an old *castrum* of which a few walls or the castle remain, rises up in the centre, on a *poype*, a relief of glacial origin. In the lower part of the plateau, ponds encircle the village, interspersed with meadows and copses. The only woods are on the edge of the cultivated fields. However, this account is not applicable to every *commune*. As one proceeds from one part of the Chalaronne to another, the territory of La Chapelle-du-Châtelard lengthens inordinately, as if it had arisen out of the union of two less important territories which were, however, more regular in form. One cannot rule out the possibility that to the former parish (now a *commune*) of La Chapelle (of Le Châtelard), mentioned from 1097 onwards, there was added the territory of Le Châtelard to the South, around a château belonging to the Archbishop of Lyons, which was surrendered in fief to Humbert of Thoire and Villars around 1200. Le Châtelard lost its status as parish in the late Middle Ages and was then absorbed into La Chapelle-du-Châtelard.[5]

The situation of Saint Guinefort's wood, where tradition has it that there was once a *castrum*, is a yet more remarkable one. The wood lies in the only enclave of the *commune* of Sandrans that is situated to the North of the Chalaronne. It is a trapezium-shaped area, 800 by 600 metres, which is inserted like a wedge between the lands of Châtillon, Romans, and La Chapelle-du-Châtelard. These lands are so interlocking at this particular spot that it is hard today, if one simply questions the inhabitants of these various villages, to know whose the wood is, for everyone claims it for his own *commune*. Can one conclude from the particular situation of this enclave that it was once densely populated, that it was abandoned and that the land was then absorbed into that of Sandrans? A cartographic study certainly implies that there was indeed, as the oral tradition gathered by

Stephen of Bourbon suggested, a *castrum* on this very site, and that it had disappeared before the middle of the thirteenth century.

Oral tradition supplies clues as to the history of abandonments which often turn out to be remarkably detailed and accurate. In fact, the abandoned fields were the object of bitter rivalries on the part of neighbouring communities. So coveted were they that interminable debates were conducted over them, and these left a lasting mark upon the collective memory.[6] Wherever possible, however, it is advisable to check these clues against the archives, by examining the surface of the soil, and by archaeological excavations. There is no visible trace of any construction in Saint Guinefort's wood. Moreover, there is not a single building or farm or chapel or even ruin in the entire enclave at Sandrans.

However, the deep ditch which crosses the hillock to the North-West, and the extremely flattened nature of this hillock, lead one to ask whether this site might not have been prepared for defensive purposes.

Between 1977 and 1980, preliminary investigations, followed by an archaeological investigation,[7] have demonstrated the artificial nature of the ditch, of the earth-works at the top of the hillock, and of the levelling of the platform. The discovery of a stake in the uppermost part of the hillock, and further to the South, the post-holes of what were clearly quite modest dwellings, may well point to the presence of a defensive site which may, on the basis of a few scattered fragments of pottery, be dated as eleventh to twelfth-century. The archaeological excavation has thus borne out the short-lived existence of a modest *castrum*, consisting of an enclosure of land, of a wood, and of a few dwellings, abandoned in the twelfth century, prior to the emergence and growth of the pilgrimage mentioned a century and a half later in Stephen of Bourbon's *exemplum*.

This excavation also uncovered, at the Southernmost edge of the platform, traces of the final phases of the pilgrimage's history. Spurred on by what informants had told us of their memories of the pilgrimage, and further encouraged by discovering large numbers of fragments of leather on the surface, just below the undergrowth, it was not long before we came upon a small pit about 0.90 metres across and 0.40 metres deep, filled with a light, blackish soil, and containing numerous fragments of children's shoes. We counted twenty soles and one complete shoe. The size of these shoes would suggest that they belonged to children one or two years old. Along with these shoes we also found numerous porcelain buttons, undoubtedly coming from woollen slippers, fragments of glass and sixty or so coins, dating from 1850 to 1919. With the exception of the oldest (a 50-centime piece from the Second Republic), the value of these coins was never higher than 5 or 10 centimes. Our discovery of this pit and of its contents, along with the oral testimony that we went on gathering throughout the period of the excavation, gave us a more precise picture of the manner in which the pilgrims' ritual actions occurred, at any rate in the second half of the nineteenth and at the beginning of the twentieth century. The pilgrims brought those of their children who were not yet able to walk, placed them briefly in the pit, where they also laid the children's shoes. The latter often bore the marks of fairly heavy use, and must therefore have belonged, in certain cases at any rate, to older children. This symbolic gesture, accompanied by the depositing of a coin of low value, was supposed to encourage the children to walk. This is clearly at variance with Stephen of Bourbon's account, and it is therefore possible that this latter form of the ritual is a fairly recent one. In fact, the pit was dug in undisturbed soil, and no older trace of the pilgrimage has been found.

The archaeological excavation has thus confirmed the preceding historical and ethnographic enquiry, and in two crucial respects. We have found that a *castrum* had indeed existed prior to the pilgrimage, just as the legend collected by Stephen of Bourbon had suggested. This discovery says much about the genesis of the legend, even if we are not concerned to uncover the 'historical truth' regarding the oral tradition, which, even in this case, cannot simply be considered as a 'mirage of reality'.[8] The material traces which have been recovered do not, to my mind, have more 'reality' than the legend collected by Stephen of Bourbon. The latter is simply one of the elements in a coherent whole which constituted the cult at a particular moment. I have not therefore allowed archaeology special privileges, though it has closed the enquiry, and may some day allow it to start all over again, nor would I want to subordinate the study of the legend to it. Rather than calling upon archaeology to tell us what 'reality' is, I would ask some equally crucial but somewhat different questions: what were the historical conditions for the production of the oral tradition? What social function is served by its obligatory reference to the past? In order to advance a reply to these questions, we must reconsider the actual content of the narrative and the social status of Stephen of Bourbon's informants.

His informants were *rustici*, who denounced the murder that the knight, the lord of the castle, had committed, and spoke of the punishment that God had inflicted upon him. They also said that they themselves, the peasants, had then reclaimed the site from the desert and had given it a religious purpose. In the very place where God had struck down a lord (*seigneur*), they established the cult of a saint for their own use.

Just as the narrative cannot be considered as a simple record of the possible existence of a *castrum* that had disappeared, so too would it be wrong to treat it as merely a reflection of the social transformations that the peasantry had undergone in the twelfth century. But it is nevertheless inseparable from them. We have little local information about these transformations, but they cannot have been so different from those that George Duby has observed in the Mâconnais nearby. A new network of villages and parishes was woven, thanks to the demographic and agricultural advances, and to the land clearances and cultivation of new fields. New power relations developed at the same time. The independent castellanies, centres of bannal seigneuries, were in danger both of becoming more dependent upon more powerful manors, and of losing their direct authority over men in favour of the small village seigneuries. The boundaries of these latter became aligned with those of the parishes, and they thus became the most effective framework for rural life. Differences in juridical status among the village population grew blurred, and social conditions became more equal. Only a small number of the richest peasants were immune from this, as also were a small group at the base, being dependents tied to the land by more than their person. The church became the centre of social life. All decisions respecting the common land which the peasants used were taken in common there, even though its possession rested ultimately with the lord. Any conflicts which arose between the lord, jealous of his rights, and the rural community, ever more confident of its strength, were also expressed in the church:

> Brought into being by the territorial seigneury, the rural community was also constructed in opposition to it. And these residential communities, which unified all the peasants of the one territory, to the exclusion of the nobles, first came into existence in the course of the twelfth century. These developments are still obscure and somewhat fleeting, for the deeds in the archives of the period, to a greater extent even than those of the tenth or thirteenth centuries, hardly mention anyone apart from the rich. Peasant life is largely absent from these accounts and one can only discern the bare outline of these forms of economic and sentimental solidarity; they begin to emerge in the following century, but will only become fully visible in the thirteenth century, when they actually confront the power of the seigneury.[9]

It was largely because the rural communities were so cohesive that they were able to achieve a partial freedom from seigneurial domination, as was also the case to the East of the Saône. Thus, in 1250, the lord of Bâgé freed the town of Bourg, its dependants and its inhabitants, and in 1253 the lord of Beaujeu followed suit and declared Miribel *libre et franc*; in 1260, Humbert of Thoire and Villars granted the men of the abbey of Chassagne, founded by his ancestors, liberty 'from all exactions, usages and other rights over the land of Villars'. A little later he also freed the men of Poncin.[10] The rural communities and seigneurs negotiated the price of these freedoms, and the latter were forced to yield to the peasants' pressure.

The original transformations that occurred in the agrarian economy of the Dombes from the thirteenth century onwards, owing to seigneurial pressure and often against the peasants' interests, provided very specific reasons for the revival and expression of these tensions. In the eleventh and twelfth centuries, some important land clearances had occurred in the area, and a varied agricultural production had arisen, as we know from the peasant dues for wheat, rye, oats, oil, honey and (particularly in the regions of Châtillon, Châtelard and Romans) wine that feature in the charters. Dues for fish are still very rare at this period. Conversely, from the thirteenth century onwards, baronial families, and the lords of Thoire and Villars in particular, set out to construct artificial ponds for their own profit, often using natural depressions which were already drained and prepared (*lescheria*). The expression *stagnum facere*, to make a pond, refers to the construction of a dike with a causeway, the digging of drainage ditches, and the submersion of adjoining fields. An undertaking of this order presupposes material resources that only the barons could mobilise. The first instances of this are mentioned from 1230 onwards (it was a pond prepared by Marguérite of Beaujeu), and it becomes more and more common during the second half of the thirteenth century. In the fourteenth century, and still more in the fifteenth century, we find a large number of pools being constructed. This allows for the establishment of a different economy, relying largely on pisciculture, one which favours the Lyonnais market nearby, and which depends upon a scattered peasant population. There is absolutely no need to account for the demographic downturn in terms of the ravages of feudal wars: 'To sum up, the feudal wars produced depopulation, depopulation produced ponds, and the ponds in their turn were a further cause of depopulation.'[11] I would argue, rather, that in this area, where abandonments were a familiar phenomenon (as Stephen of Bourbon's *exemplum* suggests), the demographic curve was affected by economic changes. A *pouillé* (list of church revenues in a diocese) tells us that, from the end of the thirteenth or the beginning of the fourteenth century, several archpriest churches in Chalamont and Sandrans were ruined (*dirute*) or left abandoned; in the latter case, the words employed (*herma* or *hermos*) may be directly linked with the place names that we have already encountered in this same zone (*silva Rimite* around 1250, *les hermitures* in 1632). This is particularly the case with the name of the church of Saint-Georges-de-Renom, one of the five parishes upon which I have focussed attention.[12] This development was not, however, unchallenged by the peasants. It was only in 1388 and 1440, admittedly, that the peasants whose fields had been flooded as a result of the digging of the new baronial ponds went so far as to break the dikes. But in 1247 a charter mentions, unfortunately without elaborating the point, the 'usages and customs' to which one had to refer in conflicts arising over the question of ponds. It was this custom that was invoked in 1388 by one Clarevallus and his men against the claims of the lady of Villars, whose two ponds had caused the fields that they owned and cultivated to be flooded.

The narrative collected by Stephen of Bourbon was formed in a climate of this sort, in which there was opposition to the power of the barons and assertiveness on the part of the peasant community. The peasants questioned by him projected the desired annihilation, by God, of the baronial *castrum* into the past, and asserted that it was they themselves who had dedicated the abandoned land to the cult. But these representations were much more than the product or the reflection of the economic, social and political changes described above. They actually contributed to the process of social transformation, and, in confronting the power of the barons, informed the class-consciousness of the peasants.

But to what community, precisely, did these peasants belong? The situation of the wood, where four or five territories meet, shows that the cult did not concern the inhabitants of a single parish. Could the site have been the object of rivalry for several adjoining communities? Unless the opposite case applied, and the cult allowed the inhabitants of five different parishes, on the borders of their respective territories, to reaffirm good neighbourly relations. This would perhaps account for the wood being situated in the territory of Sandrans, which was both the most ancient parish (known since the tenth century) and the one upon which the others depended, for it had archpriest status. If the parish was the crucial framework for social life, it is possible that inter-parish relations were cemented at the next level up in the hierarchy of ecclesiastical districts.

The wood and the legendary image of the vanished *castrum* were thus situated at the very centre of this inter-parish network, and on the borders of all these territories. I should dearly like to have been able to show how, in the nineteenth century at any rate, religious life revolved around this central point, and to reconstruct the route taken by processions, to identify all the country chapels and the placing of all the calvaries, which are now mostly destroyed. But these collective practices, and even their material traces, have completely disappeared, and my enquiry therefore stops short at that point.

But we can assume that Saint Guinefort's wood did receive women from several different parishes. One of these women at any rate, the *vetula*, was custodian of a medical and ritual knowledge. Many ('multe mulieres') were bearers of the oral tradition, which spoke of the history of the whole community. The difficulties which Stephen of Bourbon had had to overcome ('inquisivi, audivi ad ultimum') in order to obtain in confession the narrative which he reproduced were not attributable, as Dr Edouard suggested, to the deafness of an old woman. It is the very nature of an oral tradition which explains the women's reluctance to submit to a relation (confession) with a stranger which was totally at odds with what is entailed by popular notions of narration. If it is true that, even in normal relations of communication, silences are central to oral tradition (one cannot just say anything, anywhere, to anyone), because they order a whole hierarchy of rights to speech and to knowledge,[13] there is all the more reason for an intrusion to be met with an all but indomitable resistance. The obstinate silence first encountered by Stephen of Bourbon was on the part of women and mothers. It is easy to see why, in this case in particular, they were the guardians of tradition, for, in guaranteeing the biological reproduction of the community, they also guaranteed, through the rite of aggregation of children snatched from the 'fauns', and through their knowledge of collective history, its ideological reproduction.

It would thus seem reasonable to compare this narrative's function, as far as the peasantry is concerned, with that of the legend of Melusine, *maternelle et défricheuse*,[14] for certain aristocratic lineages in the twelfth century. In the same context of ideological assertion, agricultural advance and demographic increase, these two legends, that of the holy greyhound and that of the woman serpent, express in a symbolic form a group's annexation of a territory and its desire for biological growth. This comparison is all the more justified in that the two groups concerned, the peasant community and the lineage of the petty aristocracy, were, along with the town, the main frameworks for the formation and working of folk culture from the eleventh to the thirteenth century.

Historical analysis of the narrative's contents confirms what the study of the cult of Saint Guinefort, and that of the diffusion of the legend of the faithful dog, has already suggested, namely, that in chronological terms the cult ensemble of Saint Guinefort's wood was established somewhere between the eleventh and the thirteenth centuries. The actual 'origins', which may well be more ancient, of the various isolated elements matter little. The main thing is to grasp the historical conditions under which the cult was established as a unity.

The genesis of the cult coincided with momentous changes in the medieval West, and in this region in particular. The narrative collected by Stephen of Bourbon refers to what are by no means the most insignificant of these changes, namely modifications in the relations between peasants and baron, alterations in the habitat and the countryside, the inscription in space of the peasant communities. But, however striking this narrative is, it is by no means unique. I have already mentioned the large number of folk traditions collected in thirteenth-century *exempla*, which present the parish church and the community of parishioners with the curé at its head. It was in the context of this new rural community, and concurrently with it, that the peasant folk culture was constituted. It was not simply a decorative, but essentially superfluous, backdrop to the rural community, for it played a vital part in its functioning. This is why the one lasted as long as the other.

The rapid rise of the cult of Saint Guinefort is in startling contrast to its apparent immobility in the period prior to the nineteenth century. Now, the consistency of ecclesiastical judgements during this same period is likewise worthy of note. Might one account, in either case, for this fixity in terms of the relative stability of the social structure up to the dawn of the industrial revolution?

The theoretical and practical implications of this question are familiar, for it requires a satisfactory definition of the feudal mode of production, which is far from being forthcoming, and a precise study of long-term (*pluri-séculaire*) regional history, which is non-existent.

There are several pointers, however.[15] The type of agriculture that was characteristic of this region, linking unproductive ponds and fields which were flooded and cultivated by turns, developed uninterruptedly, from the thirteenth to the beginning of the nineteenth century. Its effects were considerable, for it led to a reduction in the cultivable area and to a transformation in the communications network and in the habitat (some-times to a quite drastic degree, with roads closed and hamlets brutally destroyed, in the seventeenth century, on the *seigneurs'* orders and then submerged beneath new ponds). The demographic consequences of this development have often been denounced. Thus, in 1704, an enquiry by the *Intendant* of the Suzerainty of the Dombes concluded that the region was ten times as populated in the Middle Ages, and that even in 1500 it had five times as many inhabitants and houses as at the beginning of the eighteenth century.[16] Even if these figures cannot be taken as gospel truth, they do at least give some indication of the feeling of desolation that this country then inspired. In addition, more and more voices were raised in favour of draining the ponds, which were said to encourage malaria. The medical balance-sheet for the nineteenth century was in fact little to be envied, and there was undoubtedly some relation between it and the survival of the healing cult at Sandrans, and the proliferation of similar cults throughout the region, a century or so earlier. In the *canton* of Châtillon, in 1842–7, with an infant mortality rate of 40 per 1000, life expectancy was twenty-three years, one month. In the five *communes* in the *canton* that had the most ponds (including La Chapelle-du-Châtelard, Romans, and Sandrans) the figure fell to eighteen years, five months. The equivalent figure for the whole of France, for this period, was thirty-five years.

The documentation regarding conscription confirms these figures. For, out of 323 called up, between 1837 and 1847, 303 were dismissed as unfit (90.71 per cent), 61 of them for their weak constitutions, 57 for lack of height, 33 for varicose veins, and 13 because their sight was bad. It was 'lack of height' which most clearly distinguished the *département* of Ain, at the national level, from the neighbouring *départements* during these years.[17]

Drainage works began in 1836. By 1886, the surface area of the ponds had been reduced from 20,000 to 8,600 hectares. This new transformation of the countryside was accompanied by crucial changes at all levels. The existence of traditional forms of cultivation was threatened by an increased concentration of landed property in the hands of the Lyonnais bourgeoisie. The medical situation, however, thanks to the retreat of malaria, had improved. The building of the railway put an end to the plateau's isolation, and so finally, in this desolate country, which had been such a repository of 'popular traditions', the disintegration of the folk culture began. Its disappearance was to be as rapid as its formation some seven or eight centuries before. It is from this period of decline, paradoxically enough, that we have the largest number of documents.

Almost all of the testimonies we have regarding the local cult of Saint Guinefort derive from representatives of the church, and thus ratify it at either end of its historical existence, at the moment when the folk culture had just established itself, and at the moment when it had begun to disintegrate. One could perhaps argue that the church grew more vigilant regarding the folk culture each time a profound alteration in the social structure threatened the existing equilibrium, and its own material and ideological supremacy in particular.

It is clear enough from this what was at stake in the conflict between the folk and ecclesiastic cultures regarding religion. Control over 'symbolic goods' – and in the present case, in particular, the relation between men and supernatural powers (God, saints, demons) – was crucial to the functioning of feudal society. In short, what our thirteenth-century *exemplum* does indicate is that religion was quite central to social relations, for it involved the three representatives of rural society, namely the peasants and, facing them, the baron and the clergy. The conflict between the peasants and the church, which claimed to define sanctity/sainthood and to serve as the obligatory intermediary between men and the beyond, was counterbalanced by an antagonism, which was defined in equally religious terms, between the baron and the peasants, who claimed to have established a pilgrimage upon the site of the seigneurial *castrum*.

The peasant narrative would thus seem to refer, albeit implicitly, to the terms of the trifunctional ideology of the dominant culture which, from the eleventh century onwards, assumed a systematic form.[18] According to this schema, the social hierarchy depended upon the reciprocal services of the *oratores*, who pray, of the *bellatores*, who wage war, and of the *laboratores*, who toil for all the others. Admittedly, this schema never described the concrete reality of social relations, which were actually far more complex. But it did nevertheless express something of the truth regarding seigneurial exploitation, which, if the many clues we have are to be taken at face value, the labourers were well aware of: the popular claims that were made at the time of the movement for the Truce of God, the peasant revolts and heresy are all evidence for this. Was there not a comparable resistance in the present case also?

The peasants would seem to have appropriated the ideology of the three functions, but in order to invert its terms and to modify its meaning very deeply. They arrogate to themselves the first function, that of religious sovereignty, since they claim to have installed a cult, and to have exclusive control over it. By doing this, they set themselves up against both the representatives of the military function (the knight of the legend, of whom they say with some satisfaction that God punished him, and the lord of Villars, who threatens to confiscate their possessions) and the representative of the church, the inquisitor, who lays claim to a monopoly over the sacred and destroys the peasant cult.

The situation was altogether different in the nineteenth century. Admittedly, when the documents speak once more of the pilgrimage of Saint Guinefort, the most noteworthy thing about the account is still the survival of the cult's main features, along with the lasting hostility of the dominant culture. The legend has, nevertheless, altered, and peasants have taken the place of the knight, which implies a definite change in social relations. Finally, it is worth noting the changes that took place in learned culture in the course of the century. A debate which had first been phrased in religious terms, and in the contemporary political context, profoundly polemical ones (could Christians have 'adored' a dog?), had turned into a historicist discourse ('from the Gauls to our own time') by the end of the nineteenth century. The clerics thus gave way to scholars. But what the debate may have gained in rigour it lost in violence, for in the nineteenth century there was no longer so much at stake. The triumph of the folklorists gave rise both to a laicisation of the learned culture and to a marginalisation of the folk culture, which had thereby become, as certain writers have put it, a beautiful corpse reduced to silence.[19] The real reason for this development is that in bourgeois society religion no longer played the vital role that it had played in the social relations of feudal society.

CONCLUSION

From the thirteenth to the nineteenth century, one and the same wood, in an obscure part of the *commune* of Sandrans, in what is now the *département* of Ain, was the object of a pilgrimage renowned for the healing of children. Their mothers, who were peasants, invoked Saint Guinefort, martyr, and the legend attached to this spot, recorded around 1250, and again in 1879, asserted that this saint was a dog. Their ritual gestures also remained almost unaltered from one period to the other, in spite of the passing centuries.

However tenuous and incomplete the documentation I have assembled, it presents three features which are particularly worthy of attention, and which may be held to justify the present study.

First, it allows us to study a specific fact of folklore across a very long stretch of time. Documents fascinating in themselves are available both to 'medievalist' historians and to specialists in contemporary folklore. But the former usually have to make do with a single text, while the latter regret the impossibility of going further back in time. The present study is, so far as I know, the first occasion upon which it has been possible, for a phenomenon of this order, and in a geographical space that is likewise limited, to join up the two ends of the chronological chain.

Moreover, it is not uncommon for the historian to complain that he has access only to the modes of thought of élites, of the tiny minority who knew how to write, or who had the power to make others do their writing for them. We are, admittedly, very ignorant of the culture of the popular classes in previous centuries. But we should guard against throwing the helve after the hatchet! There are many more documents from the Middle Ages than is commonly supposed, and after the fashion of Stephen of Bourbon's *exemplum*, these still await proper study a century or so after their discovery. It is not so much the documents that are lacking as the conceptual instruments necessary to understand them. But we should have the grace to acknowledge that, as much for its richness as for its precision, the document that has served as the basis for this book is a genuinely exceptional one.

Finally, if there is no lack of writings that have transmitted medieval legends, or of texts which describe ritual practices, Stephen of Bourbon's *exemplum* gives us a totally unprecedented opportunity to attend to *both* a legend *and* a folk rite. This was an almost unheard-of piece of luck, if one considers how uncommon it is even in the aristocratic culture. It is rarely, for instance, that the texts which inform us of the dubbing of knights also give us some description of the rites and legendary narratives which accompanied it. It is advisable, then, not to dissociate legend and rite, to reverse the sort of approach that has been adopted up to now. A narrowness of theoretical stance (historians of literature are not interested in legend, folklorists have only been conscious of rites), and ideological presuppositions (how could one admit that the pilgrims revered a dog–saint? The legend must then have had nothing to do with the rite) have together prevented the document from ever being considered as a coherent whole. I have tried, on the other hand, to study the two constitutive elements of the cult at the same time, and in relation to each other. Their unity, which is quite apparent in the thirteenth century, is in fact confirmed in the nineteenth century, when the legend was still attached to the cult site, while the rite, almost unaltered, was still performed there. The one did not really disappear before the other, even if evidence concerning the legend in the last century is less common than descriptions of the rite. The two remained inseparable, right until the end. It was therefore crucial to study them together, as two distinct but complementary modes of expression of the same culture. I did not therefore consider the legend as the 'origin' of the rite, even if that is how it presents itself, nor did I treat the rite as an enactment of the legend. What I have tried to clarify is the logic of their combined functioning, in order, finally, to try and understand them.

In fact, in trying to make sense of this document, I have maintained the clearest possible distinction between analysis and explanation. If one does not distinguish between these two approaches, one is condemned, under cover of what are supposedly interpretations, to paraphrase the actual documents. In the present case, the separate analysis of the diverse elements which constitute the ensemble studied took up the first three parts of this book. These elements have recovered their coherence and their historical significance in the final part.

My approach has also been characterised by an emphasis on the complementary nature of several disciplines which have too often been kept apart, namely history, folklore, ethnology, archaeology, iconography, etc. But I did not therefore succeed in resolving all the difficulties that such an approach entails; they were sometimes even aggravated, because the instruments involved had been developed in other theoretical contexts, and were therefore ill adapted to my requirements. It is something of a paradox that a structural study of narratives still depends, for research into their sources, upon the traditional history of literature, wherein a concern with 'origins' and 'influences', indeed an exclusive preoccupation with aesthetic judgements and psychologising pseudo-explanations, has for too long prevailed. The catalogues of Aarne and Thompson (amongst others), however precious they may be for the study of oral traditions, do not enable us to apprehend the logic that links the various 'motifs', or what 'possible narratives' determine the genesis and transformations of 'types'. Thanks to Van Gennep and Sébillot in France, to Hoffmann-Krayer and Bächtold-Stäubli in Germany, and to many other folklorists, the traditional approaches to folklore are now apparently easier for us to take. But in fact the historian, in the case of Van Gennep in particular, comes up against the absence of a historical perspective. What is one to make of the present state of studies in hagiography, for which we have at our disposal, thanks to the labour of the Bollandists, a prodigious mass of documents with no other index than that of the saints' names? Just think what services a Stith Thompson of hagiography might render!

These obstacles, along with many others, may partly explain the halting and somewhat flawed nature of our research. We have sought to alleviate these difficulties by adopting as rigorous an approach as possible to the methods in use. These methods were as follows:

The legend and rite described in Stephen of Bourbon's *exemplum* were first given a structural analysis, the only kind capable of accounting for the specific formal, structural and semantic qualities of the legend, inasmuch as it is treated as one of a series of adjoining and mutually illuminating narratives. This was also the only method that might help us to understand the logic of the rite, and to identify its different phases. Above all, this method enabled us to grasp the overall coherence of the document, the unity of the legend and the rite.

A second method consisted in combining ethnographic enquiry, however limited, with a study that is more familiar to the historian, that of the documents from the past. Admittedly, we arrived 'in the field' too late to see the pilgrimage in action. But it is nevertheless the case that only a minute study of the cult's spatial organisation, on the site itself, and through maps and the cadastral survey, and by interviewing inhabitants, enabled us to understand the social function of the pilgrimage in the peasant communities of centuries past.

The third method involved archaeology. In fact, our initial hypothesis did not require any archaeological prospecting, for was it not customary for a legendary castle to be represented as having been on the borders of adjoining territories? What is more, it accords here with the ideological function of a narrative in which the self-assertion of the peasants required that there be the ruin of a seigneurial castle. I have rejected out of hand the idea of trying to establish, *a priori*, the element of 'historical truth' in the legend, for a legend is clearly as 'real' as a ruin. However, research in other places has shown that oral traditions often retain a memory of actual abandonments, and in the present case examination of the shape of fields on the map makes such an abandonment seem highly probable. In fact, the excavation undertaken gives us good reason to suppose that the site was actually occupied and abandoned in the eleventh to twelfth centuries, and this is one more argument in favour of the general conclusions I have advanced as to the genesis of the cult.

Finally, the historian's traditional methods have not been neglected either. I have made particular use of onomastics and etymology, both of which offer more in the way of hypothesis than of certainty, but which, when handled with care, have enabled me to fill in the gaps in the 'popular etymology'.

If I have concentrated upon a thirteenth century document, it is not because I hold that its great age makes it any more authentic than if the cult's origins had been nearer to us in time, but because there is no more recent document that is as coherent. This is undoubtedly attributable to the rigour of the inquisitorial procedure. Efficiency and precision in the instruments of repression go together, which, as I would be the first to admit, presents a golden opportunity for the historian!

The aim of the pilgrimage was to recover the child who had been stolen by the demons of the forest, and to render to them, in exchange, their own child, the changeling, whom they had substituted for the child of a man. This restitution occurred out of the mother's sight, through a rite of passage consisting of three successive phases, namely, separation, marginality and incorporation. The intermediate situation of the cult site, half way between the *castrum* and the *silva*, was appropriate for the rite's function. A legend was, moreover, attached to this site, which for the peasants was their actual history. For they said that they themselves, upon the site of a seigneurial *castrum* that had disappeared by the 'will of God', had converted a desert into a place of pilgrimage, in order that they might there venerate as a saint and martyr the dog which had been slain as a wild beast by its master. There was thus a homology of structure between the transformations in the status of the hero of the legend and the representation of the site's history.

This narrative structure is all the more striking in that it unfolds at the same pace as that at which the peasants narrated their own history. The peasants had their own history too, for which oral tradition, in the absence of writing, was the support, and which was for them a means of collective identification. I have been struck, as much in the thirteenth-century peasant narrative, which refers to a vanished *castrum*, as in the seventeenth-century notary's deed, which mentions the former presence of chapels, as in nineteenth-century testimonies, which revive this same tradition, by the persistence of this obligatory reference to the past. Even if one were to suppose that a *castrum*, and subsequently some chapels, had existed on this spot, the real meaning of this reference to the past would still lie elsewhere. It expresses the will of the peasant community to inscribe itself within a history which would be no more neutral than the dominant one. This is clear enough in the thirteenth century, for while the rite served to guarantee the group's future (by saving children and reincorporating them into the society of men), the legend legitimised the existence of this community by exhuming, from the past, the memory of its supernatural election. Indeed, it is 'by divine will' that the lord was punished for his misdeed, and conversely it is the peasants who, out of a desert, made a consecrated place. The peasants had the conviction of being actors in a history willed by God. Their representations, their gestures and their ritual speech were all founded upon the notion *gesta Dei per paganos*.

But they were not the only persons to be active in the religious domain. The peasants may well have accused a legendary lord of having made a martyr of his dog, but conversely, the lords of Villars threatened to confiscate the 'idolators'' goods, and at the request of a Dominican inquisitor too, who was the representative of a church that held itself to be the obligatory intermediary between God and men. Hence a clerical interpretation of the cult which completely reversed its meaning, for the peasant rite was intended to drive back the dominion of evil, but the inquisitor saw it as depending upon a complicity between women and demons.

These documents have thus shown themselves to be of far more interest than one could have imagined at the start, for they both give us some insight into the class-consciousness of the peasantry and demonstrate the profoundly religious nature of ideological conflicts in feudal society.

But this interpretation gives rise to the following objection, namely, that the role of women was crucial both to the performance of the rite and to the narration of the legend. Does this contradict the claim that the ideology of the whole community found expression in this cult? Ought we not rather to conceive of it as an exclusively feminine cult, and one that had been driven out to the edges of the community's territory by the possibly more orthodox and masculine religion of the village church? This second interpretation may well provide a more convincing explanation of the cult in its later stages, but in the thirteenth century, the role of the mothers would not seem to me to have been the sign of a cultural marginality. For they were fulfilling their responsibilities with regard to the biological reproduction of the group, and also with regard to the maintenance of the community's oral traditions. Moreover, their narrative, far from speaking exclusively of women, stresses the civilising role of the whole peasantry (*homines rusticani*).

If, for the reasons stated above, Stephen of Bourbon's *exemplum* takes pride of place in our study, it should be obvious that the whole set of documents ought nevertheless to be considered as a single unit, so crucial was the long stretch of time to our understanding. Many aspects of the thirteenth century documents would have remained obscure had we not had recourse to more recent information (with respect to location, in particular) and conversely, the legend associated with the pilgrimage would not have been sought in the nineteenth century, had the medieval *exemplum* not informed us of its existence. Gaps in the documentation prevent us from tracing the cult's history in any detail, and force us to acknowledge, across seven centuries, a whole series of differences which we cannot properly explain. But we know of everything that remained unchanged, and it was this that was essential, namely the situation of the cult, the link between legend and rite, most of the ritual gestures, the main actors (mothers, children, and the *vetula* as well, whose latterday equivalent was la Fanchette Gadin). But the differences are significant too: in the legend, the knight has been replaced by a couple of farmers or a woodcutter. The medieval rite's ambiguities (cure/substitution/infanticide) have been dissipated, and it is now simply a question of curing. But some doubt has now arisen as to the saint's identity, for the nineteenth century oral tradition still has it that he is a dog, whereas the crude statuettes that were manufactured upon several occasions represent him as a man. Finally, the ultimate phase of the ritual, immersion in the river, has gone, even though the coherence of the cult ensemble depended upon it. But there is nothing arbitrary about this disappearance, for it may perhaps be attributed to the disappearance of the local belief in changelings and of a rite of substitution whose efficacy had therefore no longer to be tested in the fast-flowing waters of the Chalaronne. Thus, even if the cult was still functioning in the nineteenth century, it was functioning very differently. What there is that is enduring in this cult's structure should not be allowed to obscure the very real changes in this structure itself. The history of folklore from the medieval period to the industrial revolution was not 'static'.

If gaps in the documentation preclude an exhaustive knowledge of this history, they are nevertheless themselves a part of the problem that has to be resolved. Indeed, the rate at which texts informing us of the folk culture were produced is itself a function of ideological domination. To be more precise, the emergence of references to folklore in written documents implies that new conflicts have broken out between folk and learned culture, which will give rise to changes in social relations as a whole. Documents only begin to speak when there is some purpose to their doing so, and whilst the long, long silence of texts does not necessarily signify the complete absence of all ideological tension during that period, it is at any rate clear that the appearance and reappearance of the cult in the documents testifies to significant changes in the balance of power between folk and learned culture in the thirteenth century first of all, and subsequently in the nineteenth century. Indeed, the folk, and more particularly the peasant culture was one of the key poles in a socially differentiated system of representations peculiar to feudal Europe. If I say *a* system, in the singular, it is because these representations clearly have something in common, namely, a reference to Christianity. Even the cult in Saint Guinefort's wood, in which some claim to have identified a survival of paganism, is evidence for the thoroughgoing penetration of Christianity into the countryside, and in one of the most characteristic of medieval forms, that of the cult of saints. But I also spoke of a *differentiated* system, in contrast to those of preliterate societies. In feudal Europe, the church was in a dominant position, owing to its mastery of writing in particular, and when faced with lay persons, most of whose culture had for so long been an exclusively oral one, it obviously held considerable temporal power (think of the drafting of charters, for instance). At the same time, in a profoundly religious society, the control of writing, i.e., of the Word of God, enabled the church to legitimise its spiritual power and its pretensions, which were in fact considerable. It claimed to have exclusive knowledge of the paths to salvation, it sought to have a monopoly over dialogue with the beyond, and to determine the criteria of sanctity, etc.

Now clerical culture was very often opposed by the folk culture, which was Christian too, whatever the 'origins' of the elements combined in it. It may have been Christian, but it often ran counter to the norms of ecclesiastic culture. It is tempting to define folk culture in purely negative terms, so that, once one had extracted from it everything that was irreducible to clerical culture, one would then have a lay culture. But the difference was not simply one of content, for it also resided in the logic of its functioning, and it is therefore vital to realise that, for the peasants, there was no contradiction between the notion of sanctity and the memory of a dog, even if the theology of the period and modern rationalism have nothing to gain from such a primitive belief system (*pensée sauvage*).

The three main actors in medieval rural society, clerics, lords, and peasants, are present in Stephen of Bourbon's *exemplum*. But there was nothing serene or egalitarian about their mutual confrontations. The church was in the dominant position, opposed with respect not only to the peasants but also to the lords, whose coercive power it might well requisition. The peasants were thus in danger of losing their goods, but on a more day-to-day basis they suffered material exploitation at the hands of the lords upon whom they were dependent. The most obvious instance of this occurs in the thirteenth century when, against the peasants' best interests, the masters of the soil flooded the fields in order to make new ponds. But one can only analyse this form of exploitation by situating it within the overall context of the specific social relations of feudal Europe, to which the power of the church and the functions of religion were so central.

Stephen of Bourbon was a representative of a church that was as powerful on the spiritual as on the temporal plane, and yet he failed. He thought that he had suppressed the pilgrimage to Saint Guinefort's wood, but this was not the case. Again, at the beginning of the nineteenth century, neither the hostility of Curé Dufournet, nor the sermons of two other priests (according to Abbé Delaigue) got the better of this 'superstitious' cult. The cult was quite impervious to such attacks, and in fact lasted as long as the folk culture itself, its long life being attributable to the structural permanence of an ideological system in which folklore played an essential, albeit a secondary, role.

The clerical and folk cultures thus disappeared together. Overall alterations in the social system succeeded where violence had failed, and there was no conqueror, but two conquered parties instead. God had just died. The 'free thinkers' and the folklorists took the place of the priests, but there was nothing left for them to do but administer the last rites to the cult of Saint Guinefort.

In Baron Raverat's day, and with the advent of the narrow-gauge railway, religion (whether clerical or 'superstitious') no longer played the central role that it had so long had in feudal Europe. This had been a slow development from the Reformation to the French Revolution, until, in the name of another truth, the religion of the church was itself cast back by the Reason of the *philosophes*, into the despised hell of 'superstition'.

APPENDIX

The topographic survey of Saint Guinefort's wood, with commentary by Jean-Michel Poisson

The place called 'Saint Guinefort's wood' is situated within the *commune* of Sandrans (Ain, Bourg-en-Bresse), on the edge of the D7 (from Châtillon-sur-Chalaronne to Marlieux), about two kilometres to the South-East of Châtillon.

The site is in the shape of a roughly triangular spur oriented in a North–South direction (with the point towards the South), measuring 200 metres by 75 metres, with its highest point being 256 metres high. This tree-covered relief is bordered on the East by an ancient mill-course which at present serves a sewage farm, where there is still, however, a small stream, on the West by a meadow, and on the South by a small field which itself flanks the road (height, 241 metres).

The topographic survey, which consists of contour lines (contour interval between curves: 0.50 metres), and which is taken from the point of the spur, highlights a series of irregularities. Running from North to South, the topography displays a ditch, a knoll, and an upper and a lower platform.[1]

1. *The ditch* (W): Isolating the point from the rest of the spur, a ditch transects the whole plateau, tapering out at its edges (length: 20 metres, width: 5 metres; depth: 2 metres). Its design, and its U-shaped outline, are still plainly visible.
2. *The knoll* (Y): Immediately to the South of the ditch, a knoll rises up above the plateau. Its northern slope follows very precisely the line of the ditch's slope. Roughly ellipsoidal in shape, it measures about 15 metres by 12 (West–East). Its summit is about 10 metres above the meadow, about 2 metres above the bottom of the ditch and about 1 metre above the upper platform. Its outline, when considered in relation to the ditch, brings to mind a *vallum* or rampart of earth composed in part of reject material from the digging of the ditch, and intended for strengthening the defences at this point.[2] Over time it has become flattened out and elongated. It might also be the ruin of a (defensive) building covered over again with humus.

   The hypothesis that this was a mound is very probably untenable, for its height and surface area are not substantial enough. We know, moreover, that the 'poypes' of the Bresse region are generally far larger than most medieval mounds.
3. *The upper platform* (Y): The upper platform is rectangular in shape (about 30 metres from North to South by 25) is the site's most important feature. It is fundamentally quite flat, its angle with respect to the horizontal does not exceed 0.50 metres (in the North–South direction), and its edges are not clearly defined. Inspection of the plan will show that the knoll (X) in fact lies on the platform, whose northern side is therefore flanked by the ditch; the length of this latter in fact corresponds to the width of the shelf (total length: 40 metres; height above the meadow: 9 metres; height above the bottom of the ditch: 1 metre; above the lower platform: 4 to 5 metres).

   If one takes its situation, shape and flatness into consideration, this area could well have been inhabited. But the terrain has not been altered in any of the obvious ways. From this one can conclude that, if there were indeed constructions here, they were built with light materials (wood, daub, etc.).

4. *The lower platform* (Z): From the edge of the upper platform, the terrain falls fairly abruptly to the surrounding countryside; this slope is fairly steep and forms, to the South, a second shelf. This surface, about 40 metres by 20 (from West to East), is not horizontal, but its slope is gentle (2 metres, running from North to South) and regular. Its axis veers towards the South-West by contrast with that of the upper platform. One cannot tell from this plan alone whether one has to do with a natural relief or with an artificial construction.

This site does therefore contain a number of artificial constructions, namely the ditch (rectilinear, with parallel edges, and of a consistent depth), the upper platform (horizontal, well defined, forming a fairly precise rectangle), and one that is very probably a construction too, the knoll or *vallum* (a fairly clear shape, placed exactly on the edge of the ditch).

However, we have encountered none of the materials or furnishings that would suggest the presence of human habitation to an archaeologist, nor does the surface of the terrain imply this either. We have noticed no stones, either in heaps or by themselves, on the surface, nor have we picked up any fragments of pottery. Only the ploughed field between the point of the spur and the road has yielded up something, namely some pieces of tile and brick, and these may well have originated elsewhere (amongst them there was, in fact, a fragment of tile that was in all likelihood 'mechanically' made).

Nevertheless, these observations do not rule out the possibility that there might have been human habitation here. Wooden constructions (which were usual in this area up until the widespread use of brick in the sixteenth century, for stone was very rare) actually leave no traces in the surface. As far as knoll X is concerned, this also suggests that a *vallum* is more probable than the trace of a building.

As far as the lower platform (Z) is concerned, even if it was never the result of a deliberate act of construction, it is possible that it had once been occupied, although lying outside the more heavily defended zone.

In the light of the above observations, this site would seem to correspond very closely to that mentioned in Stephen of Bourbon's *exemplum*, where it is called a *castrum*. However, the surface area of the upper platform is very small (25 metres by 40) for a fortified *bourg*. I should be inclined, rather, to think that the term *castrum*, as used by the inquisitor, refers simply to the site's form,[3] with it comprising very few structures apart from the seigneurial *domus*. One cannot, however rule out the possibility of a community having existed here beside a sort of 'strong house'[4] (perhaps on the lower platform, or to the North of the ditch, or again 'in the open').

Commentary on the cadastral surveys

It is worth commenting upon the enclave that the *commune* of Sandrans forms at this point within those of La Chapelle-du-Châtelard and Romans, upon the passage it offers close to the boundaries of the different cantons, and upon the fact that the site is at an equal distance from the nearest centres. All these points have been considered in the main body of the text, but I should also like to make some observations in the light of the cadastral surveys (1811 and 1936).

1. The small-holdings system on the site of Saint Guinefort's wood, in the 1811 cadastral survey (does this imply a very ancient occupation of the land?); these small-holdings have largely disappeared from the new survey.
2. The successive displacements of the road (D7). Thus, the 1811 survey shows one track as a continuous line (in use at the time) and one as a dotted line (an earlier track); the 1836 one gives a third line (the present road). The tracks of roads fluctuated quite dramatically up to the middle of the nineteenth century. However, given that the displacement of the road never exceeds 500 metres at this point, there was clearly a thoroughfare between the point of the spur and the Chalaronne. Can we deduce from this that the site overlooked a thoroughfare? It would be interesting, in this respect, to know how important the Thoissey–Ambérieu road was in the Middle Ages.

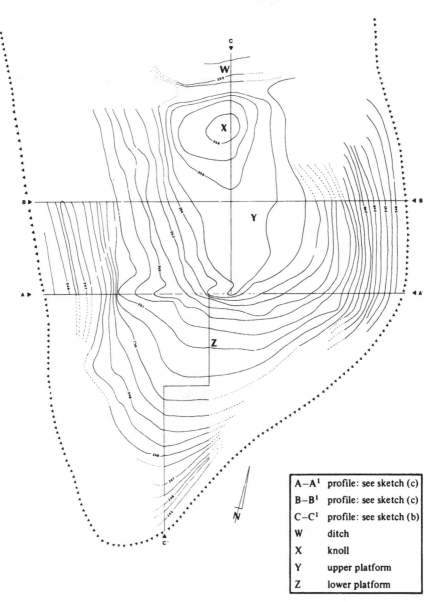

Sketch (a) The obstructed spur: topographic plan

A–A[1]	profile: see sketch (c)
B–B[1]	profile: see sketch (c)
C–C[1]	profile: see sketch (b)
W	ditch
X	knoll
Y	upper platform
Z	lower platform

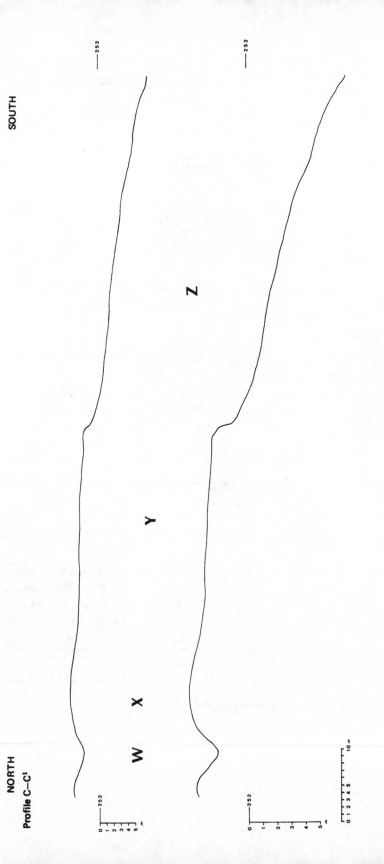

Sketch (b) North-South profile

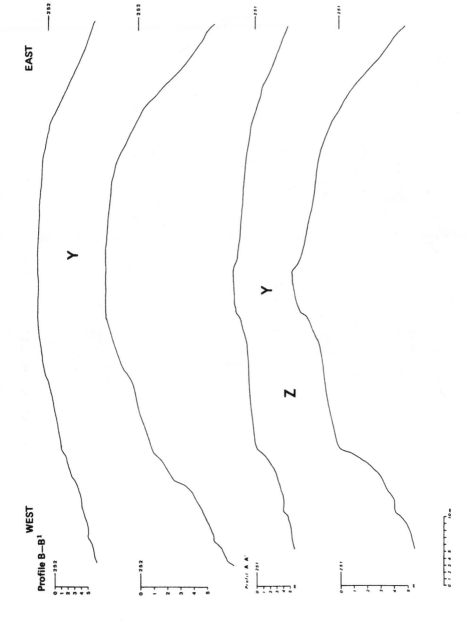

Sketch (c) West-East profile

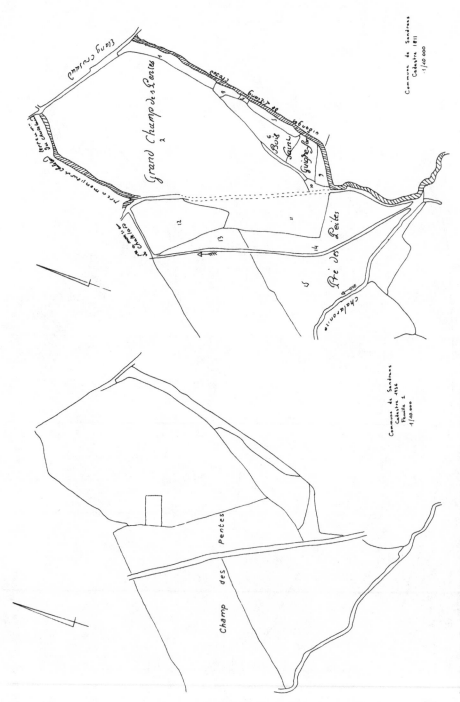

Sketch (d) Two cadastral surveys, made in 1811 and 1936

Commune de Sandrans
Cadastre 1811
·1/10 000

Commune de Sandrans
Cadastre 1936
Feuille 1
1/10 000

Étang Cruzille

Grand Champ des Pentes

Bois Sacri

Pré des Pentes

Champ des Pentes

NOTES

For abbreviations used, see Bibliography, p. 203.

Introduction

1   H. Grundmann, 'Literatus–illiteratus. Die Wandlung einer Bildungsnorm vom Altertum sum Mittelalter', *Archiv für Kulturgeschichte*, 40 (1958), 1–65.

2   On this, see the articles collected in J. Le Goff (ed.), *Time, Work and Culture in the Middle Ages*, trans. Arthur Goldhammer (Chicago and London, 1980), pp. 153–289, which provide the basis for an assessment of the change in attitudes between the early Middle Ages and the twelfth century. According to Keith Thomas, in his *Religion and the Decline of Magic* (London, 1971), the distance between the two only increased in the late medieval and early modern period. The primary works in this period are those by Carlo Ginzburg and Natalie Zemon Davis listed in the bibliography.

3   The manuscript used is the oldest known manuscript of Stephen of Bourbon's work: Bibl. Nat. MS. lat. 15, 970, fols 413ᵛ–414ʳ. I have checked the transcription in A. Lecoy de la Marche, *Anecdotes historiques, légendes et apologues tirés du recueil inédit d'Etienne de Bourbon, dominicain du XIIIᵉ siècle* (Paris, 1877), pp. 325–8, against the manuscript, a procedure which entailed only one, insignificant, correction. In addition, I have reinserted the title, which is written in the margin of the manuscript, alongside the third sentence, and which Lecoy de la Marche had omitted. This title may admittedly not be by Stephen of Bourbon, but the work of a copyist or even a user of the manuscript. Before Lecoy de la Marche, the Dominicans J. Quétif and J. Echard published the legend of the holy dog Guinefort from the same manuscript, in *Scriptores ordinis praedicatorum* (Paris, 1719–21, reprinted, 2 vols, 1910–14). J. P. Migne, in his *Encyclopédie théologique*, 2 vols (Paris, 1846–8), vol. 1, cols 780–2, quoted the text in 1846. However, neither of these publications reached such a large scholarly audience as the 1877 edition.

4   It is only fair to point out that this concern with an overall interpretation is also evident in two recent articles by V. Edouard, 'L'énigme du bois de Saint-Guinefort', *Visages de l'Ain*, 61 (May–June 1962), 26–32; and 'Le mystère de Saint-Guinefort', *Annales de l'Académie de Mâcon* (1970–1), 77–90.

5   This was an investigation by the Centre de Recherches Historiques, and a research seminar at the Ecole des Hautes Études en Sciences Sociales, devoted to the literature of *exempla* from the thirteenth to the fifteenth century, led by Jacques Le Goff and myself. One of the aims of this investigation was to produce a complete edition of Stephen of Bourbon's treatise.

6   I have done this in part in J-C. Schmitt, ' "Religion populaire" et culture folklorique', *Annales E.S.C.* (1976), 941–53.

7   This is the conclusion reached by V. Edouard.

185

Part 1: The inquisitor

1: Stephen of Bourbon

1   Most recently in J. Berlioz, 'Etienne de Bourbon, O.P. († 1261), *Tractatus de diversis materiis predicabilibus* (Troisième partie, *De dono scientie*), étude et édition', thesis for the Ecole Nationale des Chartes, 4 vols mimeographed (Paris, 1977).

2   H-C. Scheeben, 'Prediger und General Prediger im Dominikanerorden im 13. Jahrhundert', *Archivum Fratrum Praedicatorum*, 31 (1961), 112–41.

3   J. Le Goff, 'Clerical culture and folklore traditions in Merovingian civilization', in *Time, Work and Culture in the Middle Ages*, pp. 153–9.

4   A. Lecoy de la Marche, *Anecdotes historiques*, p. 292.

2: On 'superstition'

1   Saint Thomas Aquinas, *In II Sent. d. 34, q. 1.*

2   A. Lecoy de la Marche, *Anecdotes historiques*, p. 192.

3   L. K. Little, 'Pride goes before avarice: social change and the Vices in Latin Christendom', *The American Historical Review*, LXXXVI, 1 (1971), pp. 16–49, has shown how pride, the chief chivalric vice, gave way to avarice as chief of the vices, a vice given prominence by the rise of the money economy and new social categories.

4   E. Benveniste, *Indo-European Language and Society*, 2 vols (London, 1973), Ch. 7, 'Religion and superstition', pp. 516–28.

5   Isidore of Seville, *Etymologiae*, cap. III: 'De haeresi et schismati', § 6 and 7, in *P.L.*, vol. 82, col. 297.

6   I am grateful to Mme Bautier for allowing me to consult the wealth of material on the word *superstitio* in the files of the Du Cange committee at the Institut de France.

7   Roger Bacon, *Opus tertium*, ed. J. S. Brewer (London, 1859), p. 46 (my italics). I am grateful to Professor Franco Alessio of Padua University for drawing this text to my attention.

8   J. Hansen, *Zauberwahn, Inquisition und Hexenprozess im Mittelalter, und die Entstehung der grossen Hexenverfolgung* (Munich and Leipzig, 1900), pp. 127ff.

9   J. C. Caro Baroja, *The World of the Witches* (London, 1964), pp. 79ff. and N. Cohn, *Europe's Inner Demons* (London, 1975).

10   Saint Augustine, *Epistola CII (ad Deogratias)*, in *P.L.*, vol. 33, cols. 370–86, especially paragraphs 18 (col. 377) and 20 (col. 378). The same expressions are used by Albertus Magnus: 'expectare aliquid a demone vel velle aliquid percipere per ipsum, semper est fidei contumelia, et ideo apostasia'. *Commentarium in L.2. Sent.*, Dist. 7 et 10, quoted in J. Hansen, *Zauberwahn*, p. 170, n. 3.

11   This still occurs in Africa. See E. E. Evans-Pritchard, *Witchcraft, Oracles and Magic Among the Azande* (Oxford, 1937).

12   Saint Thomas Aquinas, *IIa–IIe, q. XCII, art. 2.*

13   A. Lecoy de la Marche, *Anecdotes historiques*, pp. 321–2.

14   J. Hansen, *Zauberwahn*, pp. 248–9. See in particular Thomas of Cobham, *Summa confessorum*, ed. F. Broomfield (Louvain and Paris, 1968), LXXXVIII, pp. 466–8.

15   *Dictionnaire de spiritualité*, vol. 2, cols 77–85, s.v. *canonisation*. See also the thesis by André Vauchez.

16   William of Auvergne, *De legibus*, cap. IV, XIV, XXVI, in *Opera omnia*, 2 vols (Rouen, 1674).

17   C. Du Cange, *Glossarium mediae et infimae latinitatis*, new edition, 10 vols (Niort, 1883), vol. 5, p. 148, s.v. *lucus*.

18   F. Gaffiot, *Dictionnaire illustré latin–français* (Paris, 1934), p. 925, s.v. *lucus*.

19   C. Clemen, *Fontes historiae religionis germanicae (fontes historiae religionum ex auctoribus graecis et latinis collectos)*, fasc. III (Berlin, 1928), pp. 8, 54–5, 70–3,

20   G. Dumézil, *Fêtes romaines d'été et d'automne suivi de Dix questions romaines* (Paris, 1975), p. 52.

21   J. Chaurand, *Fou, dixième conte de la vie des Pères* (Geneva, 1871).

22   A. Maury, *Croyances et légendes du Moyen Age*, new edition (Paris, 1896), pp. 9ff.

23   K. Ziegler and W. Sontheimer, *Der kleine Pauly*, 5 vols (Stuttgart, 1967), vol. 2, pp. 521–2, s.v. *faunus*.

24   J. Le Goff, 'Clerical culture', in *Time, Work and Culture*.

25   Saint Augustine, *De civitate Dei*, XV, 23: 'Silvanos et faunos quos vulgo incubos vocant.'

26   C. Du Cange, *Glossarium*, III, p. 424, s.v. *fauni* and p. 394, s.v. *fadus*.

27   William of Auvergne, *De universo*, II, 3, cap. III and cap. VIII, in *Opera omnia*, pp. 1019 and 1029.

28   Gervase of Tilbury, *Otia imperiala*, ed. G. W. von Leibniz, 2 vols, Scriptores Rerum Brunsvicensium, I (Hanover, 1707), pp. 881–1004; II, *Emendationes et supplementa* (Hanover, 1709), pp. 751–84; see especially pp. 897–8.

29   Saint Jerome, in *P.L.*, vol. 23, cols 23–4.

30   P. Sébillot, *Le Folklore de la France*, 4 vols (Paris, 1904–7), vol. 1, pp. 160–232, vol. 2, p. 92, vol. 3, pp. 114–15, vol. 4, pp. 30, 219.

31   N. Cohn, *Europe's Inner Demons*, plates 1, 2 and 4.

32   J. Le Goff, 'Ecclesiastical culture and folklore in the Middle Ages: Saint Marcellus of Paris and the dragon', in *Time, Work and Culture*, pp. 159–89.

33   J. Hansen, *Quellen und Untersuchungen zur Geschichte des Hexenwahns und der Hexenverfolgung im Mittelalter* (Bonn, 1901), pp. 38–9.

34   *Actes du Syndde d'Arras*, in *P.L.*, vol. 142, col. 1271.

35   F. Graus, *Volk, Herrscher und Heiliger im Reich der Merovinger. Studien zur Hagiographie des Merovingerzeit* (Prague, 1965), pp. 184–90.

36   F. Graus, *Volk, Herrscher und Heiliger*, p. 105. See also E. Salin, *La Civilisation mérovingienne*, 4 vols (Paris, 1949–59).

37   C. Clemen, *Fontes historiae*, pp. 54–5.

38   Burchard of Worms, *Decretum*, in *P.L.*, vol. 140, col. 835.

39   Sulpicius Severus, *Vie de saint Martin*, ed. J. Fontaine, 3 vols (Paris, 1967–9) vol. 2, pp. 1–15, p. 277. I have added the key Latin words to J. Fontaine's translation for the purposes of comparison with the text of the *exemplum*.

40   C. Clemen, *Fontes historiae*, p. 43. E. Salin, *La Civilisation mérovingienne*, vol. 4, pp. 482–3, n. 287.

41   H. Hennet de Bernoville, *Mélanges concernant l'évêché de Saint Papoul* (Paris, 1863), pp. 197–228. On the activities of the bishop, see V. Chomel, 'Pélérins languedociens au Mont-Saint-Michel', *Annales du Midi*, LXX (1958), pp. 230–9.

3: Preaching, confession, inquisition

1   H. C. Scheeben, 'Prediger und General Prediger', pp. 115–120. In 1235, for example, 'Nullus frater predicet aut *confessiones audiat* sine speciali licentia prioris sui.' At the end of the century 'Nullus autem . . . nec *predicet populo* nec confessiones extraneorum audiat sine licentia prioris sui . . .' (my italics).

2   Humbert of Romans, *De eruditione praedicatorum libri duo*, in M. de la Bigne,

Maxima bibliotheca veterum patrum, vol. 25 (Lyons, 1677), I, cap. XLIII, 'De auditu confessionum a praedicatoribus', p. 455.

3   Thomas of Cobham, *Summa confessorum*, p. 263.

4   Bibl. Nat., MS fr. 13314, fol. 9. See J. Longère, *Oeuvres oratoires de Maîtres parisiens au XII* siècle*, 2 vols (Paris, 1975), vol. 1, pp. 205–6, and II, p. 157, n. 42. And, primarily, M. Zink, *La Prédication en langue romane avant 1300* (Paris, 1976), pp. 343–4.

5   C. Chabaneau, 'Sermons et préceptes religieux en langue d'oc du XII* siècle', *Revue des Langues Romanes*, 18 (1880), p. 142. See M. Zink, *La Prédication*, pp. 354–5.

6   A. de La Borderie, ed., *Oeuvres françaises d'Olivier Maillard. Sermons et poèmes* (Nantes, 1877), pp. 95–6. See H. Martin, *Les Ordres mendiants en Bretagne* (vers 1230 – vers 1530) (Paris, 1975), p. 329.

7   H. Hennet de Bernoville, *Mélanges*, p. 225.

8   Humbert of Romans, *De eruditione praedicatorum*, vol. 2, cap. XCIX, 'Ad mulieres pauperes in villulis', p. 505.

9   Bibl. Nat., MS. lat. 17509, fol. 144ᵛ, 'Sermo ad viduas et continentes'. The *exempla* quoted have been extracted from this sermon and published separately in J. F. Crane (ed.), *The Exempla or Illustrative Stories from the Sermones Vulgares of Jacques de Vitry*, new edition (Nendeln and Leichtenstein, 1967), pp. 110–13 and 245–51 (nos. CCLXII to CCLXX).

10   Burchard of Worms, *Decretum*, in *P.L.*, vol. 140, cols 834–7, and C. Vogel, 'Pratiques superstitieuses au début du XI* siècle d'après le *Corrector sive medicus* de Burchard, évêque de Worms (965–1025)', in *Mélanges E. R. Labande* (Poitiers, 1974), pp. 751–61.

11   Alan of Lille, *Liber penitentialis*, ed. J. Longère, 2 vols (Louvain and Lille, 1965), vol. 2, pp. 118–20.

12   Thomas of Cobham, *Summa confessorum*, pp. 466–87.

13   A. Lecoy de la Marche, *Anecdotes historiques*, pp. 293–4 and 140.

14   C. Douais, *L'Inquisition, ses origines, sa procédure* (Paris, 1906), p. 284: 'Item injungantur sacerdotibus quod *in poenitentiis* diligenter inquirant hereticis . . .' (my italics). See P. M. Gy, 'Le précepte de la confession annuelle (Latran IV, c. 21) et la détection des hérétiques. S. Bonaventura et S. Thomas contre S. Raymond de Peñafort', *Revue des Sciences Philosophique et Théologique*, LVIII (1974), pp. 444–50.

15   Humbert of Romans, *De eruditione praedicatorum*, II, cap. 54 to 62.

16   *Dictionnaire de théologie catholique*, VII, 2, s.v. *inquisition*, col. 2035.

17   A. Lecoy de la Marche, *Anecdotes historiques*, pp. 229, 254, 273, 319, 322.

18   *Ibid.*, p. 261.

19   The same applied in Upper Ariège at the beginning of the fourteenth century, where *terra* was used to designate seigneurial boundaries as opposed to small families' family holdings. See E. Le Roy Ladurie, *Montaillou, village occitan de 1294 à 1324* (Paris, 1975), p. 432.

20   *Dictionnaire de théologie catholique*, s.v. *inquisition*, col. 2016. The help of the secular authorities was sought by the inquisitors in 1184 under the pontificate of Lucius III.

21   Nicolau Eymerich and Francisco Pena, *Le Manuel des Inquisiteurs*, ed. L. Sala-Molins (Paris and The Hague, 1973), p. 231.

22   The records have been published. See E. Philipon, *Dictionnaire topographique* (Paris, 1911), pp. 106 and 464–5; Valentin-Smith and M.-C. Gigne, *Bibliotheca dumbensis ou Recueil des chartes, titres et documents pour servir à l'histoire des*

Dombes, 2 vols (Trévoux, 1854–5), vol. 2, pp. 34–6, 64–5, 104–5; L. Aubert, *Mémoires pour servir à l'histoire des Dombes*, 3 vols (Trévoux, 1868), vol. 1, pp. 278, 325, 333ff., 392ff., 457, 459, 480, 497.

23   *Dictionnaire de théologie catholique*, s.v. *inquisition*, col. 2032.

24   *Bullarium ordinis praedicatorum*, vol. 1 (Rome, 1729), p. 388, and J. Hansen, *Quellen und Untersuchungen*, pp. 1–2.

25   J. Hansen, *Quellen und Untersuchungen*, p. 43.

26   Bernard Gui, *Manuel de l'Inquisiteur*, ed. and trans. G. Mollat, 2 vols (Paris, 1926).

27   A. Lecoy de la Marche, *Anecdotes historiques*, pp. 149–50.

28   J. Sprenger and M. Institaris, *Malleus maleficarum*, trans. M. Summers (London, 1928, repr. 1948).

29   A. Lecoy de la Marche, *Anecdotes historiques*, p. 322.

30   *Ibid.*, p. 299.

31   E. Le Roy Ladurie, *Montaillou*, p. 581.

32   J. Guiraud, *Histoire de l'Inquisition au Moyen Age*, 2 vols (Paris, 1935–8), vol. 2, p. 216.

33   A. Lecoy de la Marche, *Anecdotes historiques*, pp. 246 and 370–1.

34   *Ibid.*, p. 231.

35   *Ibid.*, pp. 287–8: the example of the *rusticus* who gives the lamb he is carrying on his back to some *truffatores* who have convinced him that it is a dog.

36   *Ibid.*, p. 231: the well-known example of the *rusticus* who was carrying a bundle of firewood at night on the slopes of Mont-Chat. The *Mesnie Hellequin* suddenly appeared and he was taken to a palace where he joined in a noble feast. Then he was shown to a bed in which lay a wonderfully beautiful lady. But in the morning he awoke, 'lying ignominiously on his bundle of wood, and soaked through'.

37   *Ibid.*, pp. 311–12.

38   See E. Flüry-Hérard, 'L'image de la femme dans les exempla, XIIIᵉ siècle', Mémoire de maîtrise, University of Paris IV, typewritten (Paris, n.d.).

39   A. Lecoy de la Marche, *Anecdotes historiques*, pp. 59–60, 202–3, 207–9, 315–16, 319–21, 345.

40   *Ibid.*, p. 179.

41   Y. B. Brissaud, 'L'infanticide à la fin du Moyen Age, ses motivations psychologiques et sa répression', *Revue Historique de Droit Français et Étranger*, 50 (1972), 229–56. On infanticide in the Middle Ages, see the work of the American 'History of Childhood' group, in particular the work of E. R. Coleman, R. C. Trexler and B. A. Kellum (see bibliography) and M. M. McLaughlin's very fine article, 'Survivors and surrogates: children and parents from the ninth to the thirteenth centuries', in L. Demause (ed.), *The History of Childhood* (New York, Evanston, San Francisco, London, 1975), pp. 101–81, esp. p. 119. See also the articles by D. Herlihy (see bibliography).

Part 2: The legend and the rite

4: The legend

1   The method employed here derives from J.-P. Vernant's *Myth and Society in Ancient Greece*, trans. Janet Lloyd (Brighton, 1979), pp. 168–85.

2   S. Thompson, *Motif Index of Folk Literature*, 6 vols (Helsinki, 1932–7), particularly B. 524, 1. 4. 1, 'Dog defends master's child against animal assailant'.

3   On the use of these concepts in medieval hagiography, see the works by A. Jolles,

M. Lüthi, H. Bausinger, and F. Graus (pp. 269ff.) and, most recently, H. R. Jauss, listed in the bibliography.

4   *Pañchatantra*, trans. and annotated by Edward Lancereau, preface by Louis Renon (Paris, 1965), pp. 315–16.

5   Pausanias, *Description of Greece*, trans. W. H. S. Jones, 5 vols, Loeb, (London, 1918), vol. 4, pp. 570–3.

6   John of Capua, *Directorium*, in L. Hervieux (ed.) *Les Fabulistes latins*, new edition, 5 vols (Paris, 1899), vol. 5, pp. 258–61.

7   J. Bédier showed, as long ago as 1893, that most of the fabliaux of the Middle Ages owed nothing to oriental narratives (which, some argued, were brought to the West as a result of the Crusades), but could be understood only in the context of Western folklore. See J. Bédier, *Les Fabliaux. Etude de littérature populaire et d'histoire littéraire du Moyen Age* (Paris 1893).

8   D. Paulme, *La mère dévorante. Essai sur la morphologie des contes africaines* (Paris, 1976).

9   *Les Sept sages de Rome*, in G. Paris (ed.), *Deux rédactions du Roman des Sept sages de Rome* (Paris, 1876), pp. XXIIIff. and XLIII.

10   *Ibid.*, pp. 1–54.

11   G. Buchner, *Die Historia Septem Sapientium nach der Innsbrucker Handschrift v.J.1342* (Erlangen and Leipzig, 1889), pp. 16–18.

12   *L'Ystoire des sept sages*, in G. Paris, *Deux rédactions*, pp. 74–9.

13   A. Mussafia, 'Beiträge zur Literatur der sieben weisen Meister', *Sitzungsberichte der Kaiser lichen Akademie der Wissenschaften. Philosophisch, Historische Klasse*, LVII, Heft I (1867), pp. 37–118.

14   H. A. Keller, *Li Romans des sept sages nach der pariser Handschrift* (Tübingen, 1836), pp. 46–55.

15   *Roman des sept sages*, in A. L. A. Loiseleur-Des longchamps, *Essai sur les fables indiennes et leur introduction en Europe*, together with *Le Roman des sept sages de Rome en prose*, ed. Le Roux de Lincy (Paris, 1838), pp. 16–21.

16   Johann Gobi, *Scala celi* (Lübeck, 1476, in folio), s.v. *femina*, fol. CXXVII a–b.

17   F. Madden, *The Old English Version of the Gesta Romanorum* (London, 1838), pp. 85–9.

18   H. Oesterley, *Gesta Romanorum* (Berlin, 1872), pp. 42–4.

19   C. Brunet and A. de Montaiglon, *Li Romans de Dolopathos* (Paris, 1856), pp. 168–78.

20   J. Pauli, *Schimpf und Ernst*, ed. J. Bolte, 2 vols (Berlin, 1924), no. 257.

21   John of Capua's work was translated into German shortly afterwards (*Das Buch der Weisheit*, between 1235 and 1325) and Spanish (*Exemplario contra los engaños y peligros del mundo*). This latter version, and an Arab version of the *Book of Kalila and Dimna*, were used by Raymond of Béziers in drawing up his *Liber Kalilae et Dimnae*, dedicated to Philip the Fair. On the intermediate Jewish and Arab work between the Pañchatantra and John of Capua, see: J. Derenbourg, *Deux versions hebraïques du livre de Kalilâh et Dimnah* (Paris, 1881), pp. 148–9, and Ibn-al-Muqaffa', *Le livre de Kalila et Dinna*, trans. André Miquel (Paris, 1957). The *Liber Kalilae et Dimnae* was also imitated in the thirteenth century by a Latin fabulist in Northern Italy, known by the name of 'Alter Aesopus'. In his fable XVI, the animal that saves the child is an ermine, not a dog: see E. Du Méril, *Poésies inedites du Moyen Age* (Paris, 1854), p. 242.

22   S. Baring-Gould, *Curious Myths of the Middle Ages* (London, 1888), pp. 134–44, and P. Saintyves, *En marge de la Légende dorée* (Paris, 1931), pp. 428–31. G. L. Kittredge, 'Arthur and Gorlagon', *Studies and Notes in Philology and Literature*, VIII (1903), p. 272.

23   A. G. B. Russel, 'The Rous' Roll', *Burlington Magazine*, XXX (1917), pp. 23–
      31, gives the Latin version of the Rous' Roll. For the English version, and the
      iconography, see C. E. Wright, 'The Rous' Roll. The English version', *The British
      Museum Quarterly*, XX, 4 (1956), 77–81, pl. XXVII.

24   This narrative was first published by Abbé Drouet de Maupertuy in 1713, with no
      indication of its provenance. Maupertuy's book was reviewed the following year in
      the *Journal des Savants* (Trévoux, 1714), p. 317, and provoked some debate
      among scholars, notably Abbé Lebeuf and President Bouhier in 1734. The debate
      is mentioned in a note in the *Intermédiaire des Chercheurs et des Curieux*, IV
      (1876), pp. 675–6. See also P. Saintyves, *En marge de la Légende dorée*,
      pp. 411–44.

25   See the work of A. Louis, particularly *L'Epopée française et carolingienne*
      (Saragossa, 1956); P. Sébillot, *Le Folklore*, IV, index s.v. 'Ganelon'; and M.
      Crampon, *Le Culte de l'arbre et de la forêt en Picardie* (Amiens and Paris, 1936),
      p. 166.

26   The same applies, unfortunately, to yet another version, brought to my notice by M.
      Audibert. In an interview for *Cahiers du Cinéma*, in 1954, the late Roberto
      Rossellini summed up the scenario of his film *Il miraculo* as follows: 'I would
      regard *Il miraculo* as an absolutely catholic work. I started with a sermon by Saint
      Bernadino of Siena, about a saint called Bonino. A peasant goes out into the fields
      with his dog and his two-year-old son. He leaves the dog and the child in the shade of
      an oak tree and sets off to work. On his return he discovers the child's throat cut, and
      teeth marks on its neck, and in his grief the father kills the dog, and only then notices
      a large snake and realises his error. Deeply aware of the injustice of what he has
      done, he buries the dog among the rocks nearby and on his tomb engraves the
      inscription: "Here lies Bonino [this was the dog's name] who was killed by the
      ferocity of man." Several hundred years go by, and a road now passes the tomb;
      travellers rest in the shade of the tree and read the inscription. Gradually they take
      to praying and asking for intercession from the unfortunate who is buried there.
      Miracles occur, so many that the local people build a fine church, with a tomb in
      order to transfer Bonino's body. Then they see that Bonino was a dog' (*Cahiers du
      Cinéma*, VII 37 (July 1954), p. 4). Unfortunately I have not been able to find any
      trace of this story in the sermons of Bernadino of Siena published at the beginning of
      the fifteenth century, nor in the collections of *exempla* that were drawn from them.
      Until more information comes to light I cannot make use of Rossellini's text. But it
      is still worth emphasising the details which are peculiar to this version. It is the only
      case where the child is actually killed by the snake; Bonino is the dog's name (like
      Ganelon, mentioned earlier), not the name of a saint which is bestowed upon the
      dog–martyr at a later date (as is the case with Guinefort). However, there is a real
      Saint Bonino as well, but he is known only because his name is mentioned in an
      epitaph dated 1 November 1626, saying that his relics are to be found, with those of
      two other martyrs, Soterius and Paulinus, in the church of Saint Gervase and Saint
      Protase in Pavia (*Acta sanctorum*, May, vol. 3, p. 456). Pure coincidence? As we
      shall see, this church is also the resting place of the body of the human Saint
      Guinefort. There is also the similarity between the name Bonino and one of the
      Italian forms of Guinefort, Boniforto. But, for the time being, I must not even
      suggest that there could be a connection between Stephen of Bourbon's *exemplum*,
      Saint Guinefort and Saint Bonino of Pavia, and the dog Bonino in this narrative, the
      origin of which would first of all have to be traced.

27   See J.-C. Schmitt, ' "Jeunes" et danse des chevaux de bois', in *La Religion
      populaire en Languedoc du XIIIe siècle à la moitié du XIVe siècle*, Les Cahiers de
      Fanjeaux, XI (Toulouse, 1976), pp. 127–158.

28   Vincent of Beauvais, *Speculum naturale* (Douai, 1627; new edition, Graz, 1964), Lib. XIX, CAP. XIV: 'De diversis generibus canum'.

29   R. Van Marle, *Iconographie de l'art profane au Moyen Age*, 2 vols (The Hague, 1931), pp. 32 and 217. E. Mâle, *L'Art religieux de la fin du Moyen Age en France*, 5 vols (Paris, 1931), V, p. 426. See also M. Clayton's marvellous *Catalogue of Rubbings and Brasses and Incised Slabs* (London, 1968). In particular, see pl. 23, where, side by side, the knight lies with his greyhound and the lady with her pug (dating from 1479).

30   Isidore of Seville, *Etymologiae*, Lib. XII, cap. IV: 'De serpentibus', in *P.L.*, vol. 82, cols 73–728.

31   Gervaise 'Le Bestiaire', ed. P. Meyer, *Romania*, I (1872), p. 433.

32   L. Dumont, *La Tarasque* (Paris, 1951); J. Le Goff, 'Ecclesiastical Culture . . .', in *Time, Work and Culture*.

33   Hugh of Saint-Victor, *De bestiis et aliis rebus*, Lib. III, cap. LIII, 'De serpentum varia natura', in *P.L.*, vol. 177, cols 14–64.

34   Isidore of Seville, *De natura rerum*, in *P.L.*, vol. 83, col. 981.

35   A. Van Gennep, *Manuel de folklore français contemporain*, 3 books in 9 vols (Paris, 1937–72), vol. 1, part 4, 2, p. 1440.

36   Hildegard of Bingen, *Physica*, Lib. VIII, cap. II, 'De quadam serpente', in *P.L.*, vol. 197, col. 1339.

37   F. McCulloch, *Medieval Latin and French Bestiaries* (Chapel Hill, 1962), pp. 170–1, and pl. VIII, fig. 4.

38   A. G. Ott, *Etude sur les couleurs en vieux français* (Paris, 1899), pp. 109–19.

39   Philip of Thaün, *Le Bestiaire*, ed. E. Walberg (Lund, 1900), pp. 89–90.

40   Vincent of Beauvais, *Speculum naturale*, Lib. II, cap. LXX, 'De generatione colorum in nubibus'.

41   *Ibid.*, Lib. VI, cap. XXXII.

42   A. Van Gennep, *Manuel de folklore*, vol. 1, part 3, 1, p. 924.

43   A. Schultz, *Das höfische Leben zur Zeit der Minnesinger*, new edition, 2 vols (Leipzig, 1889), vol. 1, p. 151, n. 2.

44   E. Benveniste, *Indo-European Language*, vol. 1, p. 314.

45   J.-C. Schmitt, 'Le suicide au Moyen Age', *Annales E.S.C.* (1976), p. 13.

46   *La Chanson de la Croisade albigeoise*, ed. and trans. from the Provençal by E. Martin-Chabot, 2 vols, Classiques de l'Histoire de la France Mediévale (Paris, 1960–1), vol. 1, pp. 165–7. See also the testimonies of: Pierre de Vaux de Cernay, *Hystoria albigensis*, ed. P. Guébin and E. Lyon, 3 vols (Paris, 1926), vol. 1, pp. 227–8, and vol. 3, p. 79; Aubri de Trois-Fontaines, *Chronica*, ed. P. Schetter-Boichorst, Monumenta Germaniae Historica, Scriptores, XXIII (Hanover, 1874), p. 892; Robert of Auxerre, *Chronicon*, ed. O. Holder-Eggel, *Ibid.*, XXVI (Hanover, 1882), p. 276. I am grateful to Mlle Michelle Bastard of the University of Toulouse-Le Mirail for pointing out this episode of the Albigensian crusade to me, and to M. Yves Castan for suggesting the hypothesis discussed here.

47   P. Sébillot, *Le Folklore*, vol. 2, p. 318. The martyrs of the Theban legion were also said to have been decapitated and thrown down a large well; see, in particular, the fine painting by Anton Woensam von Worms (Cologne, around 1475) in the possession of the Bayerische Staatsgemäldesammlungen at Munich, currently on loan to the Washington National Gallery.

48   *Ibid.*, vol. 1, pp. 235–6 and 349–50.

49   V. J. Propp, 'L'albero magico sulla tomba. A proposito dell'origine della fabia di magia', in V. J. Propp (ed.), *Edipo alla luce del folklore* (Turin, 1975), p. 36. In this essay, he is already pursuing the concerns he develops in *Le radici storiche dei*

racconti di fate (Turin, 1972), which, unlike the 1929 *Morphology of the Folktale* (2nd edition, Austin and London, 1968), are heavily influenced by the demands of Zhdanovism. His evolutionism, in particular, seems a little questionable nowadays. But Propp's great merits have not been sufficiently recognised: he wanted to escape the limitations of morphological analysis and argued the need for historical interpretation as well; he compared European and preliterate folklore; and he linked folktales with rituals. Besides the *Morphology*, his essays on the historical interpretation of folklore remain fundamental for any serious consideration of oral traditions.

50 F. Graus, *Volk, Herrscher und Heiliger*, p. 100, n. 267.

51 A. Lecoy de la Marche, *Anecdotes historiques*, pp. 261–6.

52 *Liber exemplorum*, no. 112, pp. 65–7; a thirteenth-century Irish *exemplum* tells of a wicked knight who constantly put off the time when he would repent. After thirty years, the earth opened up and swallowed his castle. A few moments later there was nothing to be seen on the level earth but a spring. This narrative must have been current in the Holy Land; a preacher there who used this *exemplum* on one occasion and expressed doubts about the story's authenticity was interrupted by a listener who reassured him, 'Brother, you can tell this *exemplum* without fear, I know the place where it happened!' On the forms that the maledictions took, see L. K. Little, 'Formules monastiques de malédiction aux IXe and Xe siècles', *Revue Mabillon*, LVIII (1970–5), pp. 377–99.

53 D. Fabre and J. Lacroix, *La Vie quotidienne des paysans du Languedoc au XIXe siècle* (Paris, 1974), p. 98.

54 P. Sébillot, *Le Folklore*, vol. 3, pp. 112–13.

5: The rite

1 P. Sébillot, *Le Folklore*, vol. 3, pp. 134, 279, 369, 381, 385, 387, 390, 403, 413, 419 and 421.

2 *Ibid.*, vol. 3, pp. 236, 279, 283, 307 and 330.

3 For the most recent estimate, see A. Lombard-Jourdan, 'Oppidum et banlieue. Sur l'origine et les dimensions du territoire urbain', *Annales E.S.C.* (1972), pp. 373–95, esp. 390–3, who gives the following comparisons: 3 Roman miles = 2 Celtic leagues = 1 French league = 4.440 kilometres.

4 Mme A. Lombard-Jourdan has suggested to me that this may be the result of a scribe's error, taking the adverb *rimatim* – 'through the split' – to be a proper name. This would fit with the general sense, as it is through the split in the trees that the child was passed and the demons were invoked. But the placing of the word in the sentence precludes this hypothesis, and I shall put forward a different solution below.

5 P. Riché, 'L'enfant dans le haut Moyen Age', in *Enfants et sociétés*, a special number of *Annales de Démographie Historique* (Paris, 1973), pp. 95–8.

6 Other evidence: in the twelfth century the illuminated capitals of Parma comparing the 'ages of the world' to the 'ages of life' show *pueritia* succeeding *infantia*. Cf. P. Ariès, *Centuries of Childhood* (London, 1962), pp. 23–4. At the same period in Flanders, the *Chronique du meurtre de Charles le Bon* (1127–8) describes the stages in the growth of the young William of Normandy as *infantulus, puer* and *juvenis fortis* successively. Mention is later made of *pueri* who are 'over seven years old' (cf. Galbert de Bruges, *Histoire du meurtre de Charles le Bon, Comte de Flandre (1127–1128)* ed. H. Pirenne (Paris, 1891), p. 82.

7 E. Le Roy Ladurie, *Montaillou*.

8 P. Ariès, *Centuries of Childhood*.

9   Ramon Lull, *Doctrine d'enfant, traduction française médiévale*, ed. A. Llinarès (Paris, 1969), pp. 205–6.

10   Ernest Jones, *Essays in Applied Psychoanalysis*, 2nd edition, 2 vols (London, 1951), pp. 22–109.

11   I found the same in the case of a rite of 'jeunes' punished by celestial fire; see J.-C. Schmitt, ' "Jeunes" et danse des chevaux de bois'.

12   P. Sébillot, *Le Folklore*, vol. 4, pp. 156–7.

13   *Ibid.*, vol. 3, pp. 412–14, and F. Renard, *Superstitions bressanes*, (Bourg, 1893), pp. 244–5.

14   P. Saintyves, 'Le transfert des maladies aux arbres et aux buissons', *Bulletin de la Société Préhistorique Française*, XV (1918), pp. 299–300; and E. Harlé, 'Chiffons sur buissons, au bord d'une source', *Ibid.*, p. 255.

15   *Acta sanctorum*, 'circumvectio et miraculi S. Taurini', August, vol. 2, p. 652, § 14.

16   Agobard of Lyons, *Liber contra insulsam vulgi opinionem de grandine et tonitruis*, in *P.L.*, vol. 104, cols 140–7.

17   Burchard of Worms, *Decretum*, in *P.L.*, vol. 140, col. 835, cap. 14, and col. 837, cap. 32.

18   G. Piaschewsky, *Der Wechselbalg* (Breslau, 1935); E. Hoffmann-Krayer and H. Bächtold-Stäubli, *Handwörterbuch des deutschen Aberglaubens*, 10 vols (Berlin and Leipzig, 1927–42), vol. 9, cols 835–64, s.v. *Welchselbalg*; A. Van Gennep, *Le Folklore du Dauphiné, Isère*, 2 vols (Paris, 1932–3), vol. 2, p. 533; P. Sébillot, *Le Paganisme contemporain chez les peuples celto-latins* (Paris, 1908), pp. 54ff.

19   P. Sébillot, *Le Paganisme*, pp. 35–8.

20   G. Piaschewsky, *Der Wechselbalg*, pp. 12–13.

21   J. F. Crane, *The Exempla*, p. 129, no. CCCVIIIa.

22   J. Hansen, *Quellen*, pp. 69 and 86.

23   P. Meyer, 'Chanjon, enfant changé en nourrice', *Romania* XXXII (1903), pp. 452–3; and J. Grimm, *Deutsche Mythologie* (1835 edition: *Anhang*, p. xlvi: 'tales pueri non generantur a demonibus sed sunt ipsimet demones . . .').

24   Caesar of Heisterbach, *Dialogus miraculorum*, ed. J. Stange 2 vols (Cologne, Bonn, Brussels, 1851), vol. 1, p. 124.

25   J. Hansen, *Zauberwahn*, p. 185.

26   Arch. Nat. J.J. 173, pièce 599, cited in F. Godefroy, *Dictionnaire de l'ancienne langue française et de tous ses dialectes du IXe au XVe siècle* (Paris, 1881–1902, new edition, 10 vols, Vaduz and New York, 1961), vol. 2, p. 54, s.v. *changon*. Letters of remission of 1427, after a quarrel: 'Icellui tirant en soy courrouçant l'appella *changon* et lui dist autres dures parolles a quoy ledit suppliant respondi qu'il n'estoit point *changon*, et qu'il greveroit et courrouceroit ledit tirant avant qu'il feust gaires de temps.'

27   This alteration in the judges' concerns is apparent by 1484, as in Henry Institoris and Jacobus Sprengler's *Malleus maleficarum*, in which changelings are not mentioned.

28   W. E. Peuckert, *Deutsche Volksglaube des Spätmittelalters* (Stuttgart, 1942), pp. 163–70.

29   B. de Gaiffier, 'Le diable voleur d'enfants', in B. de Gaiffier (ed.), *Etudes critiques d'hagiographie et d'iconologie*, Subsidia Hagiographica, 43 (Brussels, 1967), pp. 169–193. This work contains a very fine iconography.

30   H. Oesterley, *Gesta Romanorum*, pp. 612–14.

31   *Bibliotheca Casinensis seu codicum manuscriptorum qui in tabulario casinensi asservantur series . . . III. Florilegium* (Monte Casino, 1877), pp. 36–8. Much more recent than this Monte Casino manuscript is the fourteenth-century one from

the Bibliotheca Ambrosiana at Milan (H 82), which hardly differs at all from the former, and which M. Bianchi has used for his study of the frescos at Lentate which are contemporary with the Frankfurt painting. Other pictorial representations inspired by the *Vita fabulosa* are rare (only five or six are known) and later in date. See *Lexikon der christlichen Ikonographie* ed. E. Kirschbaum, then W. Braunfels, 8 vols (Rome, Frieburg, Basel, Vienna, 1968–76), vol. 8, col. 398.

32   K. Thomas, *Religion and the Decline of Magic*, p. 218; R. Mandrou, *Magistrate et sorciers en France au XVIIIe siècle* (Paris, 1968), pp. 102–3.

33   P. Sébillot, *Le Paganisme*, pp. 51–3.

34   O. Dobiache-Rojdestvensky, *La Vie paroissiale en France au XIIIe siècle d'après les actes épiscopaux* (Paris, 1911), pp. 60–2.

35   E. Le Roy Ladurie, *Montaillou*, pp. 578–9.

36   D. Fabre and J. Lacroix, *La Vie quotidienne*, p. 98.

6: The unity of the narrative

1   J. Le Goff, *La Civilisation de l'Occident médiéval* (Paris, 1964), p. 357.

2   E. Le Roy Ladurie, *Montaillou*, pp. 311 and 314.

3   In *Enfants et sociétés*.

4   J. Le Goff, 'Petits enfants dans la littérature des XIIe – XIIIe siècles', in *Enfants et sociétés*, pp. 129–32.

5   See, in particular, the versions of the *exemplum* called 'the hermit and the angel', which was the subject of the research seminar on *exempla*. Cf. F.-C. Tubach, *Index exemplorum* (Helsinki, 1969), no. 2558; and, among others, A. Lecoy de la Marche, *Anecdotes historiques*, p. 349. On the 'enfant gêneur', an obstacle to salvation, see also J. Le Goff, 'Entre l'enfant Jésus et les petites filles modèles', *Les Nouvelles Littéraires*, 2562 (9–16 December 1976), p. 17.

6   J. Batany, 'Regards sur l'enfance dans la littérature moralisante', in *Enfants et sociétés*, pp. 123–7.

Part 3: Saint Guinefort

7: The other cult sites

1   Passio beati Guiniforti Martyris', *Acta sanctorum*, August, vol. 5, pp. 524–30, and 'Miracula B. Guniforti martyris', *Analecta bollandiana*, XLIII (1925), pp. 359–62. See also the article 'Winifortus MS. Ticini', in *Bibliotheca hagiographica Latina*, 8590; and, lastly V. Noe's article, 'Guiniforto Santo', in *Bibliotheca sanctorum*, ed. F. Caraffa and G. Morelli, introduction by P. Ariaci, 13 vols (Rome, 1961–70), cols 527–8.

2   'Pauli Historia Longobardorum', Lib. VI, 15, in Monumenta Germaniae Historica, Scriptores rerum langobardicarum et italicarum saec. VI–IX (Hanover, 1878), p. 166.

3   J.-N. Biraben, *Les Hommes et la peste en France et dans les pays européens et méditerranéens*, vol. 2, *Les Hommes face à la peste* (Paris and The Hague, 1976), pp. 76–82.

4   For everything concerning the cult at Pavia see R. Maiocchi, *La leggenda e il culto di S. Guniforto Mart. in Pavia* (Pavia, 1917).

5   *Ibid.*, p. 152. The curé was Jean Moukel, 'Curé of Méoties' (?).

6   A. Moiraghi, *San Guniforto Mart. Notizie e preghiere* (Pavia, 1916).

7   *Vita parrochiale, parrochia dei SS. Gervasio e Protasio* (Pavia, September 1966).

8   R. Maiocchi, *La leggenda*, pp. 149–50.

9   A. Bernard and A. Bruel, *Recueil des chartes de l'abbaye de Cluny*, 6 vols (Paris, 1876–1903), vol. 4, p. 3596.

10   M. Marrier, A. Duchesne, *Bibliotheca cluniacensis*, new edition (Brussels and Paris, 1915), p. 1639.

11   *Vies des saints et des bienheureux selon l'ordre du calendrier avec l'historique des fêtes*, by the R. R. P. P. Benedictines of Paris, 13 vols (Paris, 1935–59), vol. 10, pp. 39–43.

12   G. Duby, *The Early Growth of the European Economy. Warriors and Peasants from the Seventh to the Twelfth Century*, trans. Howard B. Clarke (London, 1974), pp. 151–4.

13   G. de Valous, *Le Monachisme clunisien des origines au XVe siècle*, 2 vols (Paris, 1935), vol. 1, p. 268. See Bernard and Bruel, *Recueil des chartes*, nos 4266, 4704 and, principally, 5037, the inventory of the priory's possessions in 1261, among which there is no mention of relics of Saint Guinefort.

14   A. Guerreau, 'La fin du comte', typewritten (Paris, 1976), starts from one of the narratives of the *De miraculis*.

15   See P. Heliot and M. L. Chastang, 'Quêtes et voyages de reliques au profit des églises françaises au Moyen Age', *Revue d'Histoire Ecclésiastique*, 59 (1964), pp. 789–822, and 60 (1965), pp. 5–32, which do not, however, mention this *circumvectio*. The narrative of it is published in the *Acta sanctorum* (August, vol. 2, pp. 650–6), after the *Vita* and the two *Historiae* of the Norman saint, part of whose relics were transferred in the early Middle Ages, first to Auvergne and then to the Jura. See J. B. Mesnel, *Les Saints du diocèse d'Evreux*, vol. 1, *Saint Taurin* (Evreux, 1914). The precious shrine of Saint Taurinus (thirteenth century), preserved at Evreux, obviously has nothing to do with the one used in the *circumvectio* under consideration here.

16   G. Jeanton, *Le Mâconnais traditionaliste et populaire*, 4 vols (Mâcon, 1920–3), vol. 2, pp. 84–6.

17   A. Callet, 'Derniers vestiges du paganisme dans l'Ain', *Revue des Traditions Populaires*, XVIII (1903), p. 503.

18   Information provided by Dr V. Edouard.

19   J. Delaigue, 'Pélerinage à Saint Guinefort (près de Châtillon-les-Dombes), *Revue de la Société Littéraire, Historique et Archéologique du Département de l'Ain*, 11–12 (November–December 1886), p. 267.

20   O. de Gissey, *Discours historique de la très ancienne dévotion à Notre-Dame-du-Puy et de plusieurs belles remarques concernant particulièrement l'histoire des évêques du Velay* (Lyons, 1627), pp. 275–7.

21   On Saint Consortia, see *Vie des saints et des bienheureux*, vol. 6, p. 352. In 1399, a catalogue of the many relics kept at Cluny mentions *'Item corpus sanctae Consortiae sine capite'*. As is usual at this date, the relics of Saint Guinefort are missing from the list. Cf. Bibliothèque Nationale, Cabinet des Manuscrits, collection Baluze, vol. 257, fol. 64c. On the cult of Saint Michael and the archangels at Cluny, see K. J. Conant, *Cluny, les églises et la maison du chef d'ordre* (Paris, 1968), pp. 93–100.

22   *L'Intermédiaire des chercheurs et curieux*, XVII (1884), p. 359.

23   L. de Nussac, 'Les fontaines du Limousin: culte, pratiques, légendes', *Bulletin Archéologique du Comité des Travaux Historiques et Scientifiques* (1897), p. 175, no. 143.

24   G. Beneut, 'Le crypte à offrande de Saint-Junien (Haute-Vienne)', *Bulletin de la Société Française de Numismatique*, 28th year, 7 (July 1973), p. 450. There is no guarantee of the antiquity of the name given to the crypt.

25   Archives of the *département* of Cher, 14 G 21. I am grateful to M. J.-Y. Ribault, director of the archives, who provided me with a copy of this document (which he himself dated, with reference to the individuals mentioned in it) and of valuable information about Saint Guinefort at Bourges and in Berry.

26   Archives of the *département* of Cher, 14 G 8. The name of Saint Guinefort is also mentioned in the litanies of Bourges, according to a manuscript of 1493. See V. Leroquais, *Les Bréviaires manuscrits des bibliothèques publiques de France*, 2 vols (Paris, 1934), vol. 1, p. 324.

27   *Voyage littéraire de deux religieux de la congrégation de Saint-Maur*, 2 vols (Paris, 1717–24), vol. 1, p. 30.

28   M. de Laugardière, 'Le culte liturgique des saints à Bourges aux XIIᵉ at XIIIᵉ siècles', *Cahiers d'Archéologie et d'Histoire du Berry*, 15 (1968), p. 15 and n. 7.

29   M. Gemahling, *Monographie de l'abbaye de Saint-Satur près Sancerre (Cher)* (Paris, 1867), p. 5.

30   J. Villepelet, *Sur les traces des saints en Berry* (Bourges, 1968), pp. 25–6.

31   G. Devailly, *Le Berry du Xᵉ siècle au milieu du XIIIᵉ* (Paris and The Hague, 1973), pp. 366ff.

32   G. Laisnel de la Salle, *Croyances et légendes du centre de la France*, preface by George Sand, 2 vols (Paris, 1875–81), vol. 1, p. 321. The mention of the date appears to be a scholarly addition. This kind of invocation was probably outside the normal pattern of the calendar.

33   Information kindly provided by M. J.-Y. Ribault. See also M.-M. Martin, *Les Grandes ombres du château de Béthune du XIᵉ au XVIIIᵉ siècle (de Gilou de Sully à Maximilien de Béthune)* (Paris, 1971), pp. 20–1.

34   J. Lebeuf, *Histoire de la ville et de tout le diocèse de Paris,* 7 vols (Paris, 1883–93), vol. 2, p. 166.

35   V. Edouard, 'Le mystère de saint Guinefort', *Annales de l'Académie de Mâcon* (1970–1), p. 85, following the *Bulletin Catholique du Canton d'Ecouen* (1923–4), a reference I have not been able to check.

36   P. Blondel, *Vies des saints du diocèse de Sens et d'Auxerre* (Sens and Auxerre, 1885), pp. 40–1, who quotes the report of the translation of 26 February 1445 from the *Martyrologie sénonais* of J. B. Driot (1657). A new translation occurred in 1746, and a final one in 1845. See A. Bureau, *L'Eglise de Malicorne et le culte de Saint Fort* (Tonnerre, 1889), pp. 38–45.

37   L. M. Duru, *Calendrier historico-bibliographique des saints du diocèse de Sens et d'Auxerre*, 2 vols (Sens, 1865), pp. 51–3.

38   Bureau, *L'Eglise de Malicorne*. There seems little evidence to support the hypothesis of a cult of Saint Guinefort at Montargis, according to M. Paul Gachéof Châteaurenard in his most helpful explanatory letter of 12 March 1975.

39   V. de Beauville, *Histoire de la ville de Montdidier*, 2 vols (Paris, 1875), vol. 2, p. 428.

40   J. Corblet, *Hagiographie du diocèse d'Amiens*, 5 vols (Paris, 1869–75), vol. 3, pp. 242–3. This is the only significant study of Saint Millefort.

41   J. Fournée, *Le Culte populaire des saints en Normandie*, vol. 1, *Etude générale* (Paris, 1973), p. 205.

42   J. Séguin, *En basse Normandie* (Paris, 1929), p. 255.

43   J. Fournée, *Le Culte populaire*, pp. 81 and 207.

44   J. Corblet, *Hagiographie*, vol. 3, pp. 242ff. See D. T. Duplessis, *Description géographique et historique de la haute Normandie*, 2 vols (Paris, 1740), p. 493.

45   Notably at Flammanville. See R. Vaultier and J. Fournée, *Enquête sur les saints protecteurs et guérisseurs de l'enfance en Normandie*, typewritten (Paris, 1953);

Supplément, typewritten (Paris, 1954), p. 20. On the saint, see *Vie des saints et des bienheureux*, vol. 7, pp. 492–4.

46   R. Vaultier and J. Fournée, *Enquête*, p. 43.

47   J. Corblet, *Hagiographie*, vol. 4, p. 705.

48   *Ibid.*, vol. 3, pp. 242ff. The stone cannot now be traced. The statue has been in the museum at Crépy-en-Valois since 1973. It should not be confused with the one of Saint Radegund (or of Saint John of Valois) which is also on display in the museum and which Dr Edouard wrongly identified as the bishop. My thanks to Mme Pierrette Scart of Crépy-en-Valois, for providing me with the photograph of the statue reproduced here and for important information about this local cult (7 December 1976).

49   H. Stein, *Dictionnaire topographique de la Seine-et-Marne* (Paris, 1954), p. 500. See also J. Lebeuf, *Histoire de la ville*, vol. 4, pp. 559–60.

50   J. Lebeuf, *Histoire de la ville*, vol. 5, p. 395.

51   C. Chastelain and M. de Saint-Allais, *Martyrologe universel* (Paris, 1823), pp. 367–9. *Vie des saints et des bienheureux*, vol. 7, pp. 614–15 (25 July).

52   P. Joanne, *Dictionnaire géographique et administratif de la France*, 3 vols (Paris, 1894), vol. 3, p. 1821.

53   F. Duine, 'Pèlerins et pèlerinages', *Revue des Traditions Populaires*, XIX (1904), p. 178. Summarised in P. Sébillot, *Le Folklore*, vol. 4, pp. 156–7.

54   E. Hamonic, 'Pèlerins et pèlerinages', *Revue des Traditions Populaires*, IV (1889), p. 166. J. M. Carlo, *ibid.*, XIII (1898), p. 100. F. Duine, *ibid.*, XV (1900), p. 614.

55   E. Delaruelle, 'La spiritualité des pèlerinages à Saint-Martin-de-Tours du Ve au Xe siècle', in E. Delaruelle (ed.), *La Piété populaire au Moyen Age*, (Turin, 1975), p. 502.

8: The ethnographic enquiry in the Dombes

1   I am grateful to Abbé P. Armand for his help in this library. It was an article of his which led me to this document (P. Armand, 'La superstition dans le pays de l'Ain en 1823–1825', *Bulletin de la Société Gorini, Revue d'Histoire Ecclesiastique et d'Archéologie Religieuse du Diocèse de Belley*, 116 (1943), pp. 12–13. On Mgr Devie, see, most recently, L. and G. Trenard, *Histoire du diocèse de Belley* (Paris, 1978).

2   J. Delaigue, 'Pèlerinage à Saint Guinefort', p. 268.

3   G. Renoud, 'Visites pastorales de 1469–1470 par Etienne de la Chassaigne, évêque suffragant. . .', *Bulletin d'Histoire et d'Archéologie du Diocèse de Belley, Publié sous les Auspices de l'Abbé Gorini*, 17 (October 1952), p. 11 for the pastoral visit to Châtillon in 1469–70; *ibid.*, 22 (April 1955), p. 26, for the visit to La Chapelle-du-Châtelard; G. Guigue, *Recueil des visites pastorales du diocèse de Lyon au XVIIe et XVIIIe siècles, I, Visites de 1613–1614* (Lyons, 1926), pp. 334–340 for pastoral visits to Châtillon and La Chapelle-du-Châtelard in 1613–1614; P. Cattin, 'Catalogue des visites pastorales de l'Ain', *Bulletin d'Histoire et d'Archéologie du Diocèse de Belley, Publié sous les Auspices de la Société Gorini*, 45–6 (1970–1), pp. 3–50, for the pastoral visits of 1469, 1470, 1613, 1655, 1771 and 1784 to Châtillon, Sandrans, La Chapelle-du-Châtelard and Romans.

4   I have consulted the statistics of the Préfecture during the Empire in G. A. C. Bossi, *Statistique générale de la France publiée par ordre de Sa Majesté l'Empereur et Roi . . . Département de l'Ain* (Paris, 1856); there is valuable and detailed information about nuptial rites and charivari in the chapter 'Usages particuliers, moeurs et habitudes' (pp. 321–6). But Saint Guinefort is not mentioned. Unfor-

tunately the files of the communes, which must have been used in drawing up the statistics for the *département*, have not been preserved in its archives, as they have in some other *départements*.

5   A. Vayssière, 'Saint Guinefort, origine, forme et object du culte rendu à ce prétendu saint dans la paroisse de Romans (Ain)', *Annales de la Société d'Emulation (Agriculture, Lettres et Arts) de l'Ain*, XII (1879), pp. 104–5.

6   J. Delaigue, 'Pèlerinage à Saint Guinefort', p. 266. The manuscript of this article, written in 1885, is now kept at the hospice at Châtillon.

7   *Ibid.*, p. 266. He is confusing Comte J.-F. Perret of Châtelard with his nephew, Charles de la Rochette, Comte de Châtelard, who succeeded him at Clerdan after his death in 1843.

8   Baron Raverat, *De Lyon à Châtillon-sur-Chalaronne, par Marlieux et le chemin de fer à voie étroite* (Lyons, 1886), p. 54.

9   A. Vingtrinier, *Etudes populaires sur la Bresse et le Bugey* (Lyons, 1902), pp. 122–3.

10   Le Tessier, 'Un culte se meurt . . . . Un culte est mort', *Bulletin de la Société des Naturalistes et Archéologues de l'Ain*, XLVII (1933), pp. 231ff.

11   This was true, for example, of Marguérite Philippe in Brittany, about 1872, some of whose stories were published by F. Luzel, in *Légendes chrétiennes de la basse Bretagne* (Paris, 1881).

9: Dog and saint

1   A. Vingtrinier, *Etudes populaires*, pp. 123ff.

2   W. von Wartburg, *Französisches etymologisches Wörterbuch, eine Darstellung des gallo-romanischen Sprachschatzes*, 23 vols (vols 4–23, Basel, 1952–70), vol. 17, pp. 582–94: old French *guigner*, used by Chrétien de Troyes, from old Frankish *wingian*, from which the German *winken*, to wink, whence *guignon*, ill-luck; to fidget, to shake one's head, etc. See also O. Bloch and W. von Wartburg, *Dictionnaire étymologique de la langue française* (Paris, 1960), s.v. *guigner*.

3   J. F. Crane, *The Exempla*, p. 97, no. CCXXXII, and pp. 229–30.

4   F. Godefroy, *Dictionnaire de l'ancienne langue française*, vol. 4, pp. 481–2, s.v. *Hoche*.

5   But I am not convinced by the last steps in these authors' arguments. Thus, according to Baron Raverat, the pilgrims fell victim to a confusion between 'saint' and 'dog' as near homonyms, which is why, having first honoured ('since the Gauls') the 'dog Guinefort', they gradually came to call him 'Saint Guinefort'. If we are to believe Dr Edouard, the peasants were not themselves responsible for the confusion, which derived instead from Stephen of Bourbon: 'The Father asked if anybody knew the story of the saint (*dou tsaint*) and an old woman who was little deaf told him that she knew the story of the dog (*dou tsiin*), an old fabliau she must have heard a mountebank or traveller telling one evening.' This hypothesis is, admittedly, ingenious, but it disregards the coherence of the legend and the rite and the continuous stretch of time during which they were associated – as late as the nineteenth century, according to Vayssière's testimony.

6   *Florence de Rome, chanson d'aventure du premier quart du XIIIᵉ siècle*, ed. A. Wallenskold, 2 vols, Société des Anciens Textes Français (Paris, 1907–9); *Ogier de Danemarche, par Raimbert de Paris, poème du XIIᵉ siècle*, ed. J. Barrois, 2 vols (Paris, 1842).

7   J. de Fouilloux, *La Vénerie et l'adolescence*, ed. G. Tilander (Karlshamm, 1967), p. 168, line 31. I have consulted all the other treatises on hunting published in the same series, but without finding anything.

8   *The Continuations of the Old French Perceval of Chrétien de Troyes, I, The First Continuation*, ed. W. Roach (Pennsylvania, 1949), lines 6201–4. See also G. Paris, 'Caradoc et le serpent', *Romania* XXVIII (1899), pp. 214–31; and G. Dumézil, *The Destiny of the Warrior*, trans. Alf Hiltebeitel (Chicago and London, 1970), pp. 144–7, which compares the story of Caradoc with the Welsh narrative of 'Math, son of Mathonwy', in the Mabinogion.

9   Lines 1451ff. quoted in F. Godefroy, *Dictionnaire*, vol. 4, p. 329, and A. Tobler and E. Lommatzsch, *Altfranzösischer Wörterbuch*, 10 vols so far published (Berlin, then Wiesbaden, 1925–75), vol. 4, p. 774, where other references are quoted.

10   E. Rolland, *Faune populaire de la France*, 13 vols (Paris, 1877–1911), vol. 4, p. 9.

11   A.-F. Pott, *Die Personennamen insbesondere die Familiennamen und ihre Entstehungsarten auch unter Berücksichtigung der Ortsnamen* (Leipzig, 1859), p. 156, s.v. *Wienert, Weinrart, Weinert*, deriving from the High German *Winihart, in Freundschaft stark* (firm in friendship); the French equivalents are Guinard and Guignard. See also M. Gottschald, *Deutsche Namenkunde* (Berlin, 1971), pp. 612–13, s.v. *Winibald, Winibert*, etc. On the names of Breton saints, see J.-A. Dulaure, *Des divinités génératrices (ou du culte du phallus chez les anciens et les modernes)*, new edition (Paris, 1905), pp. 211–12; and P. Saintyves, 'Les saints protecteurs', *Revue des Traditions Populaires*, XXXI (1916), pp. 77–84: the root *guen*, which in Breton means 'white' or 'blessed', must obviously be connected with 'Guinefort', which has been recorded in Brittany. Finally, regarding the onomastics of the *chansons de geste* (Guinehart, Guinehot, Guineman), see E. Langlois, *Table des noms propres* (Paris, 1904), p. 311.

12   Stuttgart, Landesbibl. Hist. fol. 415, Martyrologium, fol. 50^r, second half of the twelfth century. For oriental representations, see *Encyclopédie universalis*, XI, s.v. *monstre*, p. 286, reproduction of a Byzantine icon from the museum of Athens; *Les Icônes dans les collections suisses*, Geneva, 14 June–29 September 1968, Musée Rath, Geneva, Musée d'Art et d'Histoire, 1968, pl. 123, a Greek icon of the eighteenth century.

13   P. Saintyves, *Saint Christophe, successeur d'Anubis, d'Hermès et d'Héraclès* (Paris, 1936).

14   G. Dumézil, *Fêtes romaines*, pp. 32–7, where the author links the word *furrinalia* with the German *Brunnen*, fountains.

15   M. Detienne, *The Gardens of Adonis*, trans. Janet Lloyd (Hassocks, Sussex, 1977), p. 9.

16   C. Cahier, *Caractéristiques des saints dans l'art populaire*, 2 vols (Paris, 1867), vol. 1, pp. 214–19. See also *Vie des saints et des bienheureux*, for the corresponding dates.

17   Jacques de Voragine, *La Légende dorée*, 2 vols (Paris, 1967), pp. 45–64.

18   *Ibid.*, pp. 11–13.

19   A. M. di Nola, *Gli aspetti magico-religiosi di una cultura subalterna italiana* (Turin, 1976), p. 31.

20   Vincent of Beauvais, *Speculum naturale* (1624 edition), Lib. XV, cap. LVI, *De canicula*, col. 1126. See also *ibid.*, Lib. XIX, cap. X–XXVII (the chapters about dogs).

21   On the medical recipes of Arnold of Villeneuve, who quotes Gilbert of England's opinions about fevers and the way they are related to the dog-days, see L. Thorndike, *A History of Magic and Experimental Science*, 2 vols (New York and London, 1923), vol. 2, p. 484, n. 9.

22   F. Godefroy, *Dictionnaire*, s.v. *cienin*, p. 122. There is no record of the word *canicule* in French before 1500.

23   V. Gay, *Glossaire archéologique du Moyen Age et de la Renaissance*, 2 vols (Paris, 1887), vol. 1, pp. 362–3, s.v. *chenet*.
24   A. Van Gennep, *Le Folklore du Dauphiné*, vol. 2, p. 351.
25   K. Thomas, *Religion and the Decline of Magic*, pp. 333–4.
26   E. Hoffman-Krayer and H. Bächtold-Stäubli, *Handwörterbuch*, vol. 8, s.v. *Stern* (*Hundstern*).
27   A. Van Gennep, *Manuel de folklore*, vol. 1, part 3, pp. 2339–67.

Part 4: Narrative time, historical time

1   M.-C. Guigue, *Topographie historique du département de l'Ain* (Trévoux, 1873), pp. 270–2.
2   *Villages désertés et histoire économique, XIᵉ–XVIIIᵉ siècles*, Ecole Pratique des Hautes Etudes, VIᵉ Section, Centre de Recherches Historiques (Paris, 1965), pp. 101–41.
3   P. Toubert, *Les Structures du Latium médiéval*, 2 vols (Rome, 1973), vol. 1, p. 359.
4   W. Janssen, *Studien zur Wüstungsfrage im frankischen Altsiedelland zwischen Rhein, Mosel und Eifelnordrand*, 2 vols (Cologne and Bonn, 1975), vol. 1, pp. 99–136.
5   M.-C. Guigue, *Notices historiques sur les fiefs et les paroisses de l'arrondissement de Trévoux* (Trévoux, 1863), p. 70; and *Essai sur les causes de la dépopulation de la Dombes* (G. Guigue, Trévoux, 1908), p. 55.
6   J. Day, 'Villagi abbandonati e tradizione orali: il caso sardo', *Archeologia Medievale*, III (1976), p. 232.
7   This archaeological investigation occupied about fifteen people under the scientific direction of Jean-Michel Poisson of the Centre Interuniversitaire d'Histoire et d'Archéologie Mediévale at Lyons. In the appendix to the book will be found the topographical description of the site before J.-M. Poisson's excavation. The exact results of the dig will be the subject of a subsequent collective publication.
8   J. Vansina, *Oral Tradition*, trans. H. M. Wright (London, 1965), especially chapter 4.
9   G. Duby, *La Société aux XIᵉ et XIIᵉ siècles dans la région mâconnaise*, new edition (Paris, 1971), p. 28.
10   Valentin-Smith and M.-C. Guigue, *Bibliotheca dumbensis*, vol. 1, pp. 6, 9, 12, 65.
11   M.-C. Guigue, *Essai sur les causes*, p. 89. Most of my data are borrowed from this very well-informed book.
12   A. Bernard, *Cartulaire de Savigny suivi du petit Cartulaire de l'abbaye d'Ainay*, 2 vols (Paris, 1853), vol. 2, pp. 922–4.
13   J. Jamin, *Les lois du silence. Essai sur la fonction sociale du secret* (Paris, 1977), p. 13.
14   J. Le Goff and E. Le Roy Ladurie, 'Mélusine maternelle et défricheuse', *Annales E.S.C.* (1971), pp. 587–622.
15   For a general idea, consult the geographers A. Demangeon, *France économique et humaine*, 2 vols (Paris, 1946–8), vol. 1, p. 85; and G. Chabot, *Géographie régionale de la France*, new edition (Paris, 1969), pp. 234–7. A useful monograph is W. Egloff, *Le Paysan dombiste* (Paris, 1937), p. 14.
16   A. Péricaud, *De l'amélioration de la Dombes, par M. de Messini* (Lyons, 1862).
17   M. Demonet, P. Dumont and E. Le Roy Ladurie, 'Anthropologie de la jeunesse masculine en France au niveau d'une cartographie cantonale (1819–1830)', *Annales E.S.C.* (1976), pp. 712–13.
18   On the Indo-European trifunctionalism studied by Georges Dumézil, and the

medieval version of it, see G. Duby, *The Three Orders: Feudal Society Imagined*, trans. Arnold Goldhammer (Chicago and London, 1981).

19   M. de Certeau, D. Julia, J. Revel, 'La beauté du mort: le concept de culture populaire', *Politique Aujourd'hui* (December 1970), pp. 3–23.

Appendix: The topographic survey of Saint Guinefort's wood

1   Cf. topographic plan.
2   Cf. profile of the spur.
3   It should be noted here that the author still speaks of a *castrum* after its destruction (line 53).
4   N.B. the presence of a *miles*.

BIBLIOGRAPHY

Abbreviations

Annales E.S.C.: Annales Economies Sociétés Civilisations
P.L.: J.-P. Migne, ed., *Patrologiae cursus completus . . . Patres ecclesiae latinae*, 221 vols. Paris, 1844–64.

Aarne, A. and Thompson, S., *The Types of Folktale. A Classification and Bibliography*, new edition. Helsinki, 1961.
Acta sanctorum, new edition, 67 vols. Paris, 1863–7.
Agobard of Lyons, *Liber contra insulsam vulgi opinionem de grandine et tonitruis*, in *P.L.*, vol. 104, cols 140–7.
Alan of Lille, *Liber penitentialis*, ed. J. Longère, 2 vols. Louvain and Lille, 1965.
Ariès, P., *Centuries of Childhood*, trans. R. Baldwick. London, 1962.
Armand, P., 'La superstition dans les pays de l'Ain en 1823–1825', *Bulletin de la Société Gorini, Revue d'Histoire Ecclésiastique et d'Archéologie Religieuse du Diocèse de Belley*, 116 (1943), 5–22.
Aubert, L., *Mémoires pour servir à l'histoire des Dombes*, 3 vols. Trévoux, 1868.
Aubri de Trois-Fontaines, *Chronica*, ed. P. Schetter-Boichorst, Monumenta Germaniae Historica, Scriptores, XXIII. Hanover, 1874.
Bacon, R., *Opus tertium*, ed. J. S. Brewer (London, 1859).
Baring-Gould, S., *Curious Myths of the Middle Ages*. London, 1888.
Bausinger, H., *Formen der Volkspoesie*. Berlin, 1968.
Beauville, V. de, *Histoire de la ville de Montdidier*, 2 vols. Paris, 1875.
Bedier, J., *Les Fabliaux. Etude de littérature populaire et d'histoire littéraire du Moyen Age*. Paris, 1893.
Beneut, G., 'La crypte à offrande de Saint-Junien (Haute-Vienne)', *Bulletin de la Société Française de Numismatique*, 28th year, 7 (July 1973), 450–4.
Benveniste, E., *Indo-European Language and Society*, trans. Elizabeth Palmer, 2 vols. London, 1973.
Berlioz, J., 'Etienne de Bourbon, O.P. († 1261), *Tractatus de diversis materiis predicabilibus* (Troisième partie, *De dono scientie*), étude et édition', thesis for the Ecole Nationale des Chartes, 4 vols mimeographed. Paris, 1977.
Bernard, A., *Cartulaire de Savigny suivi du petit Cartulaire de l'abbaye d'Ainay*, 2 vols. Paris, 1853.
Bernard, A. and Bruel, A., *Recueil des chartes de l'abbaye de Cluny*, 6 vols. Paris, 1876–1903.
Bernard Gui, *Manuel de l'Inquisiteur*, ed. and trans. G. Mollat, 2 vols. Paris, 1926.
Bibliotheca Casinensis seu codicum manuscriptorum qui in tabulario casinensi asservantur series . . . III. Florilegium. Monte Casino, 1877.
Bibliotheca sanctorum, ed. F. Caraffa and G. Morelli, introduction by P. Ciriaci, 13 vols. Rome, 1961–70.
Biraben, J.-N., *Les Hommes et la peste en France et dans les pays européens et méditerranéens. I. La Peste dans l'histoire*. Paris, 1975. *II. Les Hommes face à la peste*. Paris and the Hague, 1976.

Bloch, O. and Wartburg, W. von, *Dictionnaire étymologique de la langue française*. Paris, 1960.

Blondel, P., *Vies des saints du diocèse de Sens et d'Auxerre*. Sens and Auxerre, 1885.

Bossi, G. A. C., *Statistique générale de la France publiée par ordre de Sa Majesté l'Empereur et Roi . . . Département de l'Ain*. Paris, 1856.

Brissaud, Y. B., 'L'infanticide à la fin du Moyen Age, ses motivations psychologiques et sa répression', *Revue Historique de Droit Français et Étranger*, 50 (1972), 229–56.

Brunet, C. and Montaiglon, A. de, *Li Romans de Dolopathos*. Paris, 1856.

Buchner, G., *Die Historia Septem Sapientium nach der Innsbrucker Handschrift v.J.1342*. Erlangen and Leipzig, 1889.

Burchard of Worms, *Decretum*, in *P.L.*, vol. 140, cols 834–7.

Bureau, A., *L'Eglise de Malicorne et le culte de Saint Fort*. Tonnerre, 1889.

Caesar of Heisterbach, *Dialogus miraculorum*, ed. J. Stange, 2 vols. Cologne, Bonn, Brussels, 1851.

Cahier, C., *Caractéristiques des saints dans l'art populaire*, 2 vols. Paris, 1867.

Callet, A., 'Derniers vestiges du paganisme dans l'Ain', *Revue des Traditions Populaires*, XVIII (1903), 496–503.

Caro Baroja, J., *The World of the Witches*, trans. Nigel Glendinning. London, 1964.

Cattin, P., 'Catalogue des visites pastorales de l'Ain', *Bulletin d'Histoire et d'Archéologie du Diocèse de Belley, Publié sous les Auspices de la Société Gorini*, 46–6 (1970–1), 3–50.

Certeau, M. de, Julia, D. and Revel, J., 'La beauté du mort: Le concept de culture populaire', *Politique Aujourd'hui* (December 1970), 3–23.

Chabaneau, C., 'Sermons et préceptes religieux en langue d'oc du XIIᵉ siècle', *Revue des Langues Romanes*, 18 (1880), 105–46; 22 (1882), 157–79; 33 (1883), 53–70 and 157–69.

Chabot, G., *Géographie régionale de la France*, new edition. Paris, 1969.

Chastelain, C. and Saint-Allais, M. de, *Martyrologe universel*. Paris, 1823.

Chaurand, J., *Fou, dixième conte de la vie des Pères*. Geneva, 1871.

Chomel, V., 'Pèlerins languedociens au Mont-Saint-Michel', *Annales du Midi*, LXX (1958), 230–9.

Clayton, M., *Catalogue of Rubbings of Brasses and Incised Slabs*. London, 1968.

Clemen, C., ed., *Fontes historiae religionis germanicae (fontes historiae religionum ex auctoribus graecis et latinis collectos*, fasc. III. Berlin, 1928.

Cohn, N., *Europe's Inner Demons*. London, 1975.

Coleman, E. R., 'L'infanticide dans le haut Moyen Age', *Annales E.S.C.* (1974: 2), 315–35.

Conant, K. J., *Cluny, les églises et la maison du chef d'ordre*. Paris, 1968.

Corblet, J., *Hagiographie du diocèse d'Amiens*, 5 vols. Paris, 1869–75.

Crampon, M., *Le Culte de l'arbre et de la forêt en Picardie. Essai sur le folklore picard*. Amiens and Paris, 1936.

Crane, J. F., *The Exempla or Illustrative Stories from the Sermones Vulgares of Jacques de Vitry*, new edition. Nendeln and Lichtenstein, 1967.

Davis, N. Z., *Society and Culture in Early Modern France*. London, 1975.

Day, J., 'Villagi abbandonati e tradizione orale: il caso sardo', *Archeologia Medievale*, III (1976), 203–39.

Delaigue, J., 'Pélerinage à saint Guinefort (près de Châtillon-les-Dombes)', *Revue de la Société Littéraire, Historique et Archéologique du Département de l'Ain*, 7–8 (July–August 1886), 155–62; 9–10 (September–October 1886), 193–9; 11–12 (November–December 1886), 265–72.

Delaruelle, E., ed., *La Piété populaire au Moyen Age*. Turin, 1975.

Demangeon, A., *France économique et humaine*, 2 vols. Paris, 1946–8.

Demause, L., *The History of Childhood*. New York, Evanston, San Francisco and London, 1975.

Derenbourg, J., *Deux versions hébraïques du livre de Kalilâh et Dimnah.* Paris, 1881.

Détienne, M., *The Gardens of Adonis: Spices in Greek Mythology*, trans. Janet Lloyd. Hassocks, Sussex, 1977.

Devailly, G., *Le Berry du Xe siècle au milieu du XIIIe.* Paris and The Hague, 1973.

Dictionnaire de spiritualité. Ascétique et mystique. Doctrine et histoire, 9 vols. Paris, 1937–75.

Dictionnaire de théologie catholique..., ed. A. Vacant and E. Mangenot, then E. Amann, 30 vols. Paris, 1935–50. *Tables générales* by B. Loth and A. Michel, 3 vols. Paris, 1951–72.

Di Nola, A. M., *Gli aspetti magico-religiosi di una cultura subalterna italiana.* Turin, 1976.

Dobiache-Rojdestvensky, O., *La Vie paroissiale en France au XIIIe siècle d'après les actes épiscopaux.* Paris, 1911.

Douais, C., *L'Inquisition, ses origines, sa procédure.* Paris, 1906.

Drouet de Maupertuy, *De la vénération rendue aux reliques des saints selon l'esprit de l'Eglise et purgée de toute superstition populaire.* Avignon, 1713.

Duby, G., *The Early Growth of the European Economy. Warriors and Peasants from the Seventh to the Twelfth Century*, trans. Howard B. Clark. London, 1974.

La Société aux XIe et XIIe siècles dans la région mâconnaise, new edition. Paris, 1971.

The Three Orders: Feudal Society Imagined, trans. Arnold Goldhammer. Chicago and London, 1981.

Du Cange, C., Glossarium mediae et infirmae latinitatis, new edition, 10 vols. Niort, 1883.

Duine, F., 'Pèlerins et pèlerinages', *Revue des Traditions Populaires*, XIX (1907).

Dulaure, J.-A., *Des divinités génératrices (ou du culte du phallus chez les anciens et les modernes)*, new edition. Paris, 1905.

Du Méril, E., *Poésies inédites du Moyen Age.* Paris, 1854.

Dumézil, G., *Fêtes romaines d'été et d'automne suivi de Dix questions romaines.* Paris, 1975.

The Destiny of the Warrior, trans. Alf Hiltebeitel. Chicago and London, 1970.

Dumont, L., *La Tarasque. Essai de description d'un fait local d'un point du vue ethnographique.* Paris, 1951.

Dumont, M., Dumont, P. and Le Roy Ladurie, E., 'Anthropologie de la jeunesse masculine en France au niveau d'une cartographie cantonale', Annales E.S.C. (1976), 700–55.

Duplessis, D. T., *Description géographique et historique de la haute Normandie*, 2 vols. Paris, 1740.

Duru, L. M., *Calendrier historico-bibliographique des saints du diocèse de Sens et d'Auxerre*, 2 vols. Sens, 1865.

Edouard, V., 'L'énigme du bois de Saint-Guinefort', *Visages de l'Ain*, 61 (May–June 1962), 26–32.

'Le mystère de saint Guinefort', *Annales de l'Académie de Mâcon* (1970–1), 77–90.

Egloff, W., *Le Paysan dombiste. Etude sur la vie, les travaux des champs et le parler d'un village de la Dombes, Versailleux (Ain).* Paris, 1937.

Enfants et Sociétés, special number of *Annales de Démographie Historique.* Paris, 1973.

Evans-Pritchard, E. E., *Witchcraft, Oracles and Magic among the Azande.* Oxford, 1937.

Eymerich, N. and Pena, F., *Le Manuel des Inquisiteurs*, ed. L. Sala-Molins. Paris and The Hague, 1973.

Fabre, D. and Lacroix, J., *La Vie quotidienne des paysans du Languedoc au XIXe siecle.* Paris, 1974.

Flüry-Hérard, E., 'L'Image de la femme dans les exempla, XIIIe siècle', Mémoire de maîtrise, University of Paris IV, typewritten, Paris, n.d.

Fournée, J., *Le Culte populaire des saints en Normandie*, vol. 1, *Etude générale.* Paris, 1973.

Gaffiot, F., *Dictionnaire illustré latin-français.* Paris, 1934.

Gaiffier, B. de, *Etudes critiques d'hagiographie et d'iconologie*, Subsidia Hagiographica Series, 43. Brussels, 1967.

Galbert de Bruges, *Histoire du meurtre de Charles le Bon, Comte de Flandre (1127–1128)*, ed. H. Pirenne. Paris, 1891.

Gay, V., *Glossaire archéologique du Moyen Age et de la Renaissance*, 2 vols. Paris, 1887.

Gemahling, M., *Monographie de l'abbaye de Saint-Satur près Sancerre (Cher)*. Paris, 1867.

Gervaise, 'Le Bestiaire', ed. P. Meyer, *Romania*, I (1872), 420–43.

Gervase of Tilbury, *Otia imperialia*, ed. G. W. von Leibniz, 2 vols, Scriptores Rerum Brunsvicensium, vol. 2. Hanover, 1707. Vol. 2, *Emendationes et supplementa*. Hanover, 1709.

Ginzburg, C., *I Benandanti. Stregoneria e culti agrari tra cinquecento e seicento*. Turin, 1966.

The Cheese and the Worms: the Cosmos of a Sixteenth-century Miller, trans. J. and A. Tedeschi. London, 1980.

Gissey, O. de, *Discours historique de la très ancienne dévotion à Notre-Dame-du-Puy et de plusieurs belles remarques concernant particulièrement l'histoire des évêques du Velay*. Lyons, 1627.

Godefroy, F., *Dictionnaire de l'ancienne langue française et de tous ses dialectes du IXe au XVe siècle*. Paris, 1881–1902; new edition, 10 vols, Vaduz and New York, 1961.

Gottschald, M., *Deutsche Namenkunde. Unsere Familiennamen nach ihren Entstehung und Bedeutung*. Berlin, 1971.

Graus, F., *Volk, Herrscher und Heiliger im Reich der Merovinger. Studien zur Hagiographie des Merovingerzeit*. Prague, 1965.

Grimm, J., *Deutsche Mythologie*, Göttingen, 1835; new edition, 3 vols, Gütersloh, 1876–8.

Grundmann, H., 'Literatus–illiteratus. Die Wandlung einer Bildungsnorm vom Altertum zum Mittelalter', *Archiv für Kulturgeschichte*, 40 (1958), 1–65.

Guerreau, A., *La Fin du comte. Esquisse d'analyse d'un récit de Pierre le Vénérable et de ses rapports avec la culture populaire et la culture savante de l'Europe féodale*, typewritten. Paris, 1976.

Guigue, G., *Recueil des visites pastorales du diocèse de Lyon aux XVIIe et XVIIIe siècles, I, Visites de 1613–1614*. Lyons, 1926.

Guigue, M.-C., *Essai sur les causes de la dépopulation de la Dombes et l'origine de ses étangs*, G. Guigue. Trévoux, 1908.

Notices historiques sur les fiefs et paroisses de l'arrondissement de Trévoux. Trévoux, 1863.

Topographie historique du département de l'Ain. Trévoux, 1873.

Guiraud, J., *Histoire de l'Inquisition au Moyen Age*, 2 vols. Paris, 1935–8.

Gy, P. M., 'Le précepte de la confession annuelle (Latran IV, c. 21) et la détection des hérétiques. S. Bonaventure et S. Thomas contre S. Raymond de Peñafort', *Revue des Sciences Philosophique et Théologique*, LVIII (1974), 444–50.

Hamonic, E., 'Pèlerins et pèlerinages', *Revue des Traditions Populaires*, IV (1889).

Hansen, J., *Quellen und Untersuchungen zur Geschichte des Hexenwahns und der Hexenverfolgung im Mittelalter*. Bonn, 1901.

Zauberwahn, Inquisition und Hexenprozess im Mittelalter, und die Entstehung der grossen Hexenverfolgung. Munich and Leipzig, 1900.

Harlé, E. 'Chiffons sur buissons, au bord d'une source', *Bulletin de la Société Préhistorique Française*, XIV (1917), 389–91, 441–3; XV (1918), 224–5, 485.

Heliot, P. and Chastang, M. L., 'Quêtes et voyages de reliques au profit des églises françaises au Moyen Age', Revue d'Histoire Ecclésiastique, 59 (1964), 789–822, and 60 (1965), 5–32.

Hennet de Bernoville, H., *Mélanges concernant l'évêché de Saint Papoul. Pages extraites et traduites d'un manuscrit du XVe siècle*. Paris, 1863.

Herlihy, D. 'Medieval children', in B. K. Lackner and K. Roy Philip (eds), *Essays on Medieval Civilization* (Austin and London, 1978), 109–41.

Hervieux, L., *Les Fabulistes latins depuis le siècle d'Auguste jusqu'à la fin du Moyen Age*, new edition, 5 vols. Paris, 1899. Vol. 5, *Jean de Capoue et ses dérivés*.

Hildegard of Bingen, *Physica*, in *P.L.*, vol. 197, cols 1117–352.

Hoffmann-Krayer, E. and Bächtold-Stäubli, H., *Handwörterbuch des deutschen Aberglaubens*, 10 vols. Berlin and Leipzig, 1927–42.

Hugh of Saint-Victor, *De bestiis et aliis rebus*, in *P.L.*, vol. 177, cols 14–164.

Humbert of Romans, *De eruditione praedicatorum libri duo*, in M. de la Bigne, ed., *Maxima Bibliotheca Veterum Patrum*, vol. 25, Lyons, 1677.

Ibn al-Muqaffa', *Le Livre de Kalila et Dimna*, trans. André Miquel. Paris, 1957.

L'Intermédiairie des chercheurs et curieux. Questions et réponses littéraires, historiques, scientifiques et artistiques. Trouvailles et curiosités, published on the 15 and 30 of each month since 1864.

Isidore of Seville, *De natura rerum*, in *P.L.*, vol. 83, cols 963–1018.

Jacques de Fouilloux, *La Vénerie et l'adolescence*, ed. G. Tilander. Karlshamm, 1967.

Jacques de Voragine, *Legenda aurea*, ed. Th. Graesse. Dresden and Leipzig, 1846.

Jacques de Voragine, *La Légende dorée*, 2 vols. Paris, 1967.

Jamin, J., *Les Lois du silence. Essai sur la fonction sociale du secret*. Paris, 1977.

Jannsen, W., *Studien zur Wüstungsfrage im frankischen Altsiedelland zwischen Rhein, Mosel und Eifelnordrand*, 2 vols. Cologne and Bonn, 1975.

Jauss, H. R., 'Littérature médiévale et théorie des genres', *Poétique*, I (1970), 79–101.

Jeanton, G., *Le Mâconnais traditionaliste et populaire*, 4 vols. Mâcon, 1920–3.

Joanne, P., *Dictionnaire géographique et administratif de la France*, 3 vols. Paris, 1894.

Johann Gobi, *Scala celi*. Lübeck, 1476, in folio.

Jolles, A., *Formes simples*. Paris, 1972.

Jones, E., *Essays in Applied Psychoanalysis*, 2nd edition, 2 vols. London, 1951.

Keller, H. A., *Li Romans des sept sages nach der pariser Handschrift*. Tübingen, 1836.

Kellum, B. A., 'Infanticide in England in the later Middle Ages', *History of Childhood Quarterly: the Journal of Psychohistory*, 1, 3 (1974), 367–88.

Kittredge, G. L., 'Arthur and Gorlagon', *Studies and Notes in Philology and Literature*, VIII (1903), 149–275.

La Borderie, A. de, *Oeuvres françaises d'Olivier Maillard. Sermons et poèmes*. Nantes, 1877.

Laisnel de la Salle, G., *Croyances et légendes du centre de la France. Souvenirs du vieux temps. Coutumes et traditions populaires comparées à celles des peuples anciens et modernes*, preface by George Sand, 2 vols. Paris, 1875–81.

Langlois, E., *Table des noms propres de toute nature compris dans les chansons de geste imprimées*. Paris, 1904.

Laugardière, M. de, 'Le culte liturgique des saints à Bourges aux XIIᵉ et XIIIᵉ siècles', *Cahiers d'Archéologie et d'Histoire du Berry*, 15 (1968), 12–17.

Lebeuf, J., *Histoire de la ville et de tout le diocèse de Paris*, 7 vols. Paris, 1883–93.

Lecoy de la Marche, A., *Anecdotes historiques, légendes et apologues tirés du recueil inédit d'Etienne de Bourbon, dominicain du XIIIᵉ siècle*. Paris, 1877.

Le Goff, J. *La Civilisation de l'Occident mediéval*. Paris, 1964.

'Entre l'enfant Jésus et les petites filles modèles', *Les Nouvelles Littéraires*, 2562 (9–16 December 1976).

Le Goff, J. (ed.), *Time, Work and Culture in the Middle Ages*, trans. Arthur Goldhammer. Chicago and London, 1980.

Le Goff, J. and Le Roy Ladurie, E., 'Mélusine maternelle et défricheuse', *Annales E.S.C.* (1971), 587–622.

Leroquais, V., *Les Bréviaires manuscrits des bibliothèques publiques de France*, 2 vols. Paris, 1934.

Le Roy Ladurie, E., *Montaillou, village occitan de 1294 à 1324*. Paris, 1975 (see also *Montaillou: Cathars and Catholics in a French Village 1294–1324*, abridged. trans. Barbara Bray, London, 1978).

Le Tessier, 'Un culte se meurt . . . Un culte est mort', *Bulletin de la Société de Naturalistes et Archéologues de l'Ain*, XLVII (1933), 231 ff.

Lexikon der christlichen Ikonographie, ed. E. Kirschbaum, then W. Braunfels, 8 vols. Rome, Freiburg, Basel, Vienna, 1968–76.

Little, L. K., 'Formules monastiques de malédiction aux IXᵉ et Xᵉ siècles', *Revue Mabillon*, LVIII (1970–5), 377–99.

'Pride goes before avarice: social change and the Vices in Latin Christendom', *The American Historical Review*, LXXVI, 1 (1971), 16–49.

Loiseleur-Deslongchamps, A. L. A., *Essai sur les fables indiennes et leur introduction en Europe*, together with *Le Roman des sept sages de Rome en prose*, ed. Le Roux de Lincy. Paris, 1838.

Lombard-Jourdan, A., 'Oppidum et banlieue. Sur l'origine et les dimensions du territoire urbain', *Annales E.S.C.* (1972), 373–95.

Longère, J., *Oeuvres oratoires de Maîtres parisiens au XIIᵉ siècle. Etude historique et doctrinale*, 2 vols. Paris, 1975.

Louis, A., *L'Epopée française et carolingienne*. Saragossa, 1956.

Lüthi, M., *Das europäische Volksmärchen. Form und Wesen*. Bern, 1947.

Luzel, F., *Légendes chrétiennes de la basse Bretagne*. Paris, 1881.

Madden, F., *The Old English Version of the Gesta Romanorum*. London, 1838.

Maiocchi, R. *La leggenda e il culto di S. Guniforto Mart. in Pavia*. Pavia, 1917.

McCulloch, F., *Medieval Latin and French Bestiaries*. Chapel Hill, 1962.

McLaughlin, M. M., 'Survivors and surrogates: children and parents from the ninth to the thirteenth centuries', in L. Demause (ed.), *History of Childhood*.

Mâle, E., *L'Art religieux de la fin du Moyen Age en France. Etude sur l'iconographie du Moyen Age et sur ses sources d'inspiration*, 5 vols. Paris, 1931.

Mandrou, R., *Magistrats et sorciers en France au XVIIIᵉ siècle. Une analyse de psychologie historique*. Paris, 1968.

Marrier, M. and Duchesne, A., *Bibliotheca cluniacensis*, new edition. Brussels and Paris, 1915.

Martin, H., *Les Ordres mendiants en Bretagne (vers 1230 – vers 1530)*. Paris, 1975.

Martin-Chabot, E. (ed. and trans.), *La Chanson de la Croisade albigeoise*, 2 vols, Classiques de l'Histoire de la France Mediévale. Paris, 1960–1.

Martin, M.-M., *Les Grandes ombres du château de Béthune du XIᵉ au XVIIIᵉ siècle (de Gilou de Sully à Maximilien de Béthune)*. Paris, 1971.

Maury, A., *Croyances et légendes du Moyen Age*, new edition. Paris, 1896.

Mesnel, J. B., *Les Saints du diocèse d'Evreux*, 2 vols. Evreux, 1914.

Meyer, P., 'Chanjon, enfant changé en nourrice', *Romania*, XXXII (1903), 452–3.

Migne, J.-P., *Encyclopédie théologique, 48. Dictionnaire des sciences occultes*, 2 vols. Paris, 1846–8.

'Miracula B. Guniforti martyris', *Analecta bollandiana*, XLIII (1925), 359–62.

Moiraghi, A., *San Guneforto Mart. Notizie e preghiere*. Pavia, 1916.

Mussafia, A., 'Beiträge zur Literatur der sieben weisen Meister', *Sitzungsberichte der Kaiserlichen Akademie der Wissenschaften. Philosophisch, Historische Klasse*, LVII, Heft I. (1867), 37–118.

Nussac, L. de, 'Les fontaines du Limousin: culte, pratiques, légendes', *Bulletin Archéologique du Comité des Travaux Historiques et Scientifiques* (1897), 150–77.

Oesterley, H., *Gesta Romanorum*. Berlin, 1872.

Ott, A. G., *Etude sur les couleurs en vieux français*. Paris, 1899.

Pañchatantra, trans. and annotated by Edouard Lancereau, preface by Louis Renon. Paris, 1965.

Paris, G., 'Caradoc et le serpent', *Romania*, XXVIII (1899), 214–31.

Deux rédactions du Roman des Sept Sages de Rome. Paris, 1876.

'Passio beati Guinforti martyris', *Acta sanctorum*, August, vol. 5, 524–30.

Patissier, J., *Les Classes populaires dans la Dombes seigneuriale (XIIIe et XIVe siècles)*. Trévoux, 1946.

Paul the Deacon, 'Historia Longobardoram', in Monumenta Germaniae Historica, Scriptores rerum longobardorum et italicarum succ. VI–IX. Hanover, 1878.

Pauli, J., *Schimpf und Ernst*. Strasbourg, B. Greininger, in folio, 1535.

Schimpf und Ernst, ed. J. Bolte, 2 vols. Berlin, 1924.

Paulme, D., *La Mère dévorante. Essai sur la morphologie des contes africains*. Paris, 1976.

Pausanias, *History of Greece*, trans. W. H. S. Jones, 5 vols, Loeb. London, 1918.

Péricaud, A., *De l'amélioration de la Dombes, par M. de Messimi*. Lyons, 1862.

Petré, H., Cantel, R. and Ricard, R., 'Exemplum'. Entry in *Dictionnaire de spiritualité*, IV, 2. Paris, 1961.

Petrus Comestor, *Historia scholastica. Liber Genesis. P.L.*, vol. 198, cols 1055–1142.

Peuckert, W. E., *Deutsche Volksglaube des Spätmittelalters*. Stuttgart, 1942.

Philipon, E., *Dictionnaire topographique du département de l'Ain comprenant les noms de lieux anciens et modernes*. Paris, 1911.

Philip of Thaün. *Le Bestiaire*, ed. E. Walberg. Lund, 1900.

Piaschewsky, G., *Der Wechselbalg. Ein Beitrag zum Aberglauben der nordeuropäischen Volker*. Breslau, 1935.

Pierre de Vaux de Cernay, *Hystoria albigensis*, ed. P. Guébin and E. Lyon, 3 vols. Paris, 1926.

Pott, A.-F., *Die Personennamen insbesondere die Familiennamen und ihre Entstehungsarten auch unter Berücksichtigung der Ortsnamen*. Leipzig, 1859.

Propp, V. J., *Edipo alla luce del folklore. Quattro studii di etnografia storico-strutturale*. Turin, 1975.

Morphology of the Folktale, 2nd edition. Austin and London, 1968.

Le radici storiche dei racconti di fate. Turin, 1972.

Quétif, J. and Echard, J., *Scriptores ordinis praedicatorum*. Paris, 1719–21; new edition, 2 vols, Paris, 1910–14.

Raimbert de Paris, *Ogler de Danemarche, par Raimbert de Paris, poème du XIIe siècle*, ed. J. Barrois, 2 vols. Paris, 1842.

Ramon Lull, *Doctrine d'enfant, traduction française médiévale*, ed. A. Llinarès. Paris, 1969.

Raverat, Baron, *De Lyon à Châtillon-sur-Chalaronne, par Marlieux et le chemin de fer à voie étroite. Etude géologique, historique et descriptive du plateau de la Dombes, son passé, son present, son avenir, avec cartes*. Lyons, 1886.

Renard, F., *Superstitions bressanes*. Bourg, 1893.

Renoud, G., 'Visites pastorales de 1469–1470 par Etienne de la Chassaigne, évêque suffragant...', *Bulletin d'Histoire et d'Archéologie du Diocèse de Belley, Publié sous les Auspices de l'Abbé Gorini*, 17 (October 1952), 1–18; 18 (April 1953), 27–31; 20 (March 1954), 15–21; 21 (September 1954), 14–22; 22 (April 1955), 19–29; 25 (August–September 1956), 1–12; 26 (April 1957), 2–13.

Riché, P. 'L'enfant dans le haut Moyen Age', in *Enfants et sociétés*.

Roach, W. (ed.), *The Continuations of the Old French Perceval of Chrétien de Troyes, I, The First Continuation*, Pennsylvania, 1949.

Robert of Auxerre, *Chronicon*, ed. O. Holder-Eggel, Monumenta Germaniae Historica, Scriptores, XXVI. Hanover. 1882.

Rolland, E., *Faune populaire de la France, noms vulgaires, dictons, proverbes, légendes, contes et superstitions'*, 13 vols. Paris, 1877–1911.

Russel, G. B., 'The Rous' Roll', *Burlington Magazine*, XXX (1917), 23–31.

Saintyves, P., *En marge de la Légende dorée; songes miracles et survivances; essai sur la formation de quelque thèmes hagiographiques*. Paris, 1931.

Saint Christophe, successeur d'Anubis, d'Hermès et d'Héraclès. Paris, 1936.

'Les saints protecteurs des nourrices et les guérisseurs de maladies des seins', *Revue des Traditions Populaires*, XXXI (1916), 77–84.

'Le transfert des maladies aux arbres et aux buissons', *Bulletin de la Société Préhistorique Française*, XV (1918), 296–300.

Salin, E., *La Civilisation mérovingienne d'après les sépultures, les textes et le laboratoire*, 4 vols. Paris, 1949–59.

Scheeben, H.-C., 'Prediger und General Prediger im Dominikanerorden im 13. Jahrhundert', *Archivum Fratrum Praedicatorum*, 31 (1961), 112–41.

Schmitt, J.-C. ' "Jeunes" et danse des chevaux de bois. Le folklore meridional dans la littérature des *exempla* (XIIIe–XIVe siècles)' in *La Religion populaire en Languedoc du XIIIe siècle à la moitié du SIV^e siècle*, Les Cahiers de Fanjeaux, XI (Toulouse, 1976), 127–58.

' "Religion populaire" et culture folklorique', *Annales E.S.C.* (1976), 941–53.

'Le suicide au Moyen Age', *Annales E.S.C.* (1976), 3–28.

Schultz, A., *Das höfische Leben zur Zeit der Minnesinger*, new edition, 2 vols. Leipzig, 1889.

Sébillot, P., *Le Folklore de la France*, 4 vols. Paris, 1904–7.

Le Paganisme contemporain chez les peuples celto-latins. Paris, 1908.

Séguin, J., *En basse Normandie. Saints guérisseurs, saints imaginaires, dévotions populaires; leur statuaire; leurs rapports avec les assemblées, les confréries, les légendes et dictons, les foires, la botanique, etc.* Paris, 1929.

Sprenger, J. and Institoris, H., *Malleus maleficarum*, trans. M. Summers. London, 1928, repr. 1948.

Stein, H., *Dictionnaire topographique de la Seine-et-Marne*. Paris, 1954.

Sulpicius Severus, *Vie de saint Martin*, ed. J. Fontaine. 3 vols. Paris, 1967–9.

Thomas, K., *Religion and the Decline of Magic*. London, 1971.

Thomas of Cobham, *Summa confessorum*, ed. F. Broomfield. Louvain and Paris, 1968.

Thompson, S., *Motif Index of Folk Literature. A classification of narrative elements in folk tales, ballads, myths, fables, medieval romances, exempla, fabliaux, jest books and local legends*. 6 vols. Helsinki, 1932–7.

Thorndike, L., *A History of Magic and Experimental Science During the first Thirteen Centuries of our Era, 2 vols. New York and London, 1923.*

Tobler, A. and Lommatzsch, E., *Altfranzösisches Wörterbuch*, 10 vols so far published. Berlin, then Wiesbaden, 1925–75.

Toubert, P., *Les Structures du Latium médiéval. Le Latium méridional et la Sabine du IXe siècle à la fin du XIIe siècle*, 2 vols. Rome, 1973.

Trenard, L. and G., *Histoire du diocèse de Belley*. Paris, 1978.

Trexler, R. C., 'Infanticide in Florence: new sources and first results', *History of Childhood Quarterly: the Journal of Psychohistory*, I, 1 (1973), 98–116.

Index Exemplorum. A Handbook of Medieval Religion Tales. Helsinki, 1969.

Valentin-Smith and Guigue, M.-C., *Bibliotheca Dumbensis ou Recueil des chartes, titres et documents pour servir à l'histoire des Dombes*, 2 vols. Trévoux, 1854–85.

Valous, G. de, *Le Monachisme clunisien des origines au XVe siècle*, 2 vols. Paris, 1935.

Van Gennep, A., *Le Folklore du Dauphiné, Isère; étude descriptive et comparée de psychologie populaire*, 2 vols. Paris, 1932–3.

Manuel de folklore français contemporain, 3 books in 9 vols. Paris, 1937–72.

Les Rites de passage, new edition. Paris, 1969.

Van Marle, R., *Iconographie de l'art profane au Moyen Age et à la Renaissance et la décoration des demeures*, 2 vols. The Hague, 1931.

Vansina, J., *Oral Tradition. A Study in Historical Method*, trans. H. M. Wright. London, 1965.

Vaultier, R. and Fournée, J., *Enquête sur les saints protecteurs et guérisseurs de l'enfance en Normandie*, typewritten. Paris, 1953. *Supplément*, typewritten. Paris, 1954.

Vayssière, A., 'Saint Guinefort, origine, forme, et objet du culte rendu a ce prétendu saint dans la paroisse de Romans (Ain)', *Annales de la Société d'Emulation (Agriculture, Lettres et Arts) de l'Ain*, XII (1879), 94–108, 209–21.

Vernant, J.-P., *Myth and Society in Ancient Greece*, trans. Janet Lloyd. Brighton, 1979.

Vies des saints et des bienheureux selon l'ordre du calendrier avec l'historique des fêtes, by the R.R. P.P. Benedictines of Paris, 13 vols. Paris, 1935–59.

Villages désertés et histoire économique, XIᵉ–XVIIIᵉ siècles. Ecole Pratique des Hautes Etudes, VIᵉ Section, Centre de Recherches Historiques, Paris, 1965.

Villepelet, J., *Sur les traces des saints en Berry*. Bourges, 1968.

Vincent of Beauvais, *Speculum naturale*. Douai, 1624; new edition, Graz, 1964.

Vingtrinier, A., *Etudes populaires sur la Bresse et le Bugey*. Lyons, 1902.

Vita parrochiale, parrochia dei SS. Gervasio e Protasio. Pavia, September 1966.

Vogel, C., 'Pratiques superstitieuses au début du XIᵉ siècle d'après le *Corrector sive medicus* de Burchard, évêque de Worms (965–1025)', in *Mélanges E.R. Labande*. Poitiers, 1974.

Voyage littéraire de deux religieux de la congrégation de Saint-Maur, 2 vols. Paris, 1717–24.

Wallenskold, A. (ed.), *Florence de Rome, chanson d'aventure du premier quart du XIIIᵉ siècle*, 2 vols, Société des Anciens Textes Français. Paris, 1907–9.

Wartburg, W. von, *Französisches etymologisches Wörterbuch, eine Darstellung des gallo-romanischen Sprachschatzes*. I, Bonn, 1929; II.1, Leipzig and Berlin, 1940; II.2, Basel, 1946; III, Paris, 1934; IV–XXIIIBasel, 1952–70.

William of Auvergne, *Opera omnia*, 2 vols. Rouen, 1674.

Wright, C. E., 'The Rous' Roll. The English version', *The British Museum Quarterly*, XX, 4 (1956), 77–81, pl. XXVI–XXVII.

Ziegler, K. and Sontheimer, W., *Der Kleine Pauly*, 5 vols. Stuttgart, 1967.

Zink, M., *La Prédication en langue romane avant 1300*. Paris, 1976.

INDEX